60

60

CHARLES CAPRARELLA

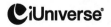

60

iUniverse books may be ordered through booksellers or by contacting:

iUniverse
1663 Liberty Drive
Bloomington, IN 47403
www.iuniverse.com
844-349-9409

ISBN: 978-1-6632-1998-5 (sc)
ISBN: 978-1-6632-1999-2 (e)

Print information available on the last page.

iUniverse rev. date: 04/21/2021

FOREWORD

"The writer does most who gives the reader the most knowledge and takes from him the least time." Sydney Smith

I have often said books can be like coaches, many use too many words, try too hard and are from a similar mold. But many get to the point, have an impact and know how to win. In this book I wanted to be in that later category, and I hope I achieved that goal. Like the above quote suggest, my goal was to deliver a story and knowledge in the simplest and quickest amount of time. I hope you will benefit from reading it.

But like the below quote postulates, there are many schools of thought, this was just mine. Question authority and always think!

"Beware of the man of one book." Saint Thomas Aquinas

INTRODUCTION

When I was 11 my father had his first heart attack. I was in the hospital room when the cardiologist came to speak with my young dad. The doctor said, "We need to perform open heart surgery and you have a 50/50 chance of survival. If you live through the operation you are going to have to stop eating eggs (he called them cardio bombs), cheeses, cut back on meats and quit smoking." This was in 1974 when open heart surgery was still in its infancy.

My dad survived surgery but hardly changed his ways. He continued to smoke cigarettes, albeit he cut back, but he kept eating the same way. He took his daily doses of "heart pills" religiously until he suffered the "big one," only 13 years later. I remember him telling me, "I am going out my way." Almost a suicide if you ask me!

I can remember first thinking about becoming a vegetarian at 12. I was watching a documentary about meat production with my dad and from that point on eating flesh just sort of grossed me out. Plus, I remembered what the doctor told my dad. I have been a vegetarian off and on since the age of 12. Not always a good practicing vegetarian but I'd say about 90% of the time. I write these words at 52.

Once I turned about 45 it became more difficult to maintain weight. I was eating more processed foods and middle-aged metabolism is not so kind. Anyway, I decided to attempt a 60 day modified fast to try and lose about 50 pounds. As I start my journey at age 52, I am 5'10" and 212 pounds.

In my life I have known the content feeling of being in top condition but in contrast, I have known what it is like to gain unwanted weight and the compromised feeling that goes along with it but for the most part I have enjoyed good health and have not been sick for many years.

I can tell you from experience that just because you become a vegetarian does not mean you will be slim and eating meat does not mean you will be overweight. It is just a matter of caloric intake vs. calories burnt, your genetic make-up and body-style. I eat too much and am addicted to food just like most of the American population.

I have read many books and studies about the benefits of a plant based-whole food-calorie restricted lifestyle but up until now, although I have tried a few times, I have not been able to stay consistent with it. So, for the next 60 days, I am going to keep a journal and keep a record of what I eat.

It has been widely known since the early 1930s that a calorie restricted diet will not only add years to your lifespan but cure sickness, increase overall stamina and perhaps save the planet from starvation.

I aim to eat less than 1200 calories a day of highly nutritional foods for the next 60 days. With that calculation I figure I should slim down to my ideal weight of 160 to 170 pounds. I am going to start out with a modified 30-day juice fast and then eat a plant based diet consisting of no more than 1200 calories a day.

Here we go!

DAY: 1
WEIGHT: 212
DATE: JULY 28, 2016

"Everything is food if you are truly hungry. Everything is poison if you are overfed." Sadhguru

It is widely known that a major step one can take to improve life is to restrict caloric intake. For a man, about 2500 calories is considered ideal and for a woman, about 1800. However, far less calories are needed to live well.

My body weight has fluctuated much of my adult life on a diet consisting mostly of plant based foods. However, I have eaten my share (more than enough) of processed high calorie foods too. But our bodies are resilient, and it is usually not too late to change.

I believe our number one addiction is food. Food is a widely accepted addiction that has been masked since childhood. "Eat your meat and drink your milk for good health," is what our parents, teachers, doctors and advertisers told us. These lies are imbedded in our subconscious mind. Therefore, it will take some time to re-program ourselves to change our thinking.

I grew up in Needham Massachusetts where I excelled at sports and ate better than most but eating too much was always emphasized in my Italian/Albanian upbringing. Everything we did involved food.

My parents were great depression survivors so perhaps them growing up with "lack" was something that they never wanted their children to experience. This coupled with the fact that food in America is so widely available made it difficult for me to eat lightly.

Most of us have the great luxury in this country to choose what we want to eat, and I realize how lucky we are. I am simply choosing to extend my life-quality by eating less calories but at the same time, eating nutrient rich foods that will benefit me. This is the first day of that journey.

Summary of food intake from day 1:

40 ounces of kale, carrot, ginger, apple and cucumber juice: 600 calories

Small salad: 300 calories

Total calories: 900

Exercise: Rode bike 12 miles and lifted some weights.

Thoughts from my bike ride: As I rode my bicycle, I kept telling myself, "You can do this."

DAY: 2
WEIGHT: 209
DATE: JULY 29, 2016

"Starvation literally means starvation. It does not mean skipping a meal or not eating for 24 hours. Or not eating for three days even. The belief that meal skipping or short-term fasting causes "starvation mode" is so completely ridiculous and absurd that it makes me want to jump out the window."
Martin Berkhan

We have all said, "I am starving," after not eating for just a few hours. We have all planned a day trip and seemed to bring enough food for an army. We seem to plan most everything we do around food. I think of how it would be a nice change to center activities around good conversation, simply existing, where food is not the star attraction. Were the burnt flesh of animals and their processed body parts are replaced with plant based foods or no food at all.

It is always nice to see that scale go down- unless of course on rare occasion, one wants it to go up. This book is for the 80% of the people in America who struggle with weight and food addiction, but it will not be for everyone.

I feel lighter today, but I woke up groggy. I have read that the first few days of a fast are the hardest, so I am not surprised. We are basically experiencing withdrawals but once you get through the first few days it becomes easier.

We are fortunate as a society to have massive food choices, but we eat too much and that is a problem. Too much eating destroys our environment, causes bloating, depression, bruised self-images, diabetes, heart disease, upset stomachs and the list goes on and on. The great news is we can easily reverse this as our bodies have the ability, unlike machines, to rejuvenate.

Many things we do seem to be associated with food. Every event, every celebration, everything! And many times, the food associated with those events are high fat, useless foods that contribute greatly to us getting sick. This thinking starts from birth, so we need to reshape our thinking.

As an example, little Sally gets ice cream when she has a sore throat. Little Billy gets cake when he does well at school. This sort of thinking must change.

Health care cost rage out of control as we stuff our faces irresponsibly and the evil advertisers trick us to eat more of their client's death foods. After all, the more we eat, the more money they make.

Summary of food intake from day 2:

32 ounces of mixed vegetable juice: 400 calories

Large salad: 400 calories

Total calories: 800

Exercise: Biked 12 miles. 25 push-ups.

Thoughts from my bike ride: *Caloric totals will be estimates based on a basic understanding of caloric content of food. Caloric content of foods will not be provided in this booklet.

Today was my birthday, turned 53 and I felt euphoric most of the day. I wasn't really all that hungry.

DAY: 3

WEIGHT: 208
DATE: JULY 30, 2016

"More die in the United States of too much food than of too little." John Kenneth Galbraith

The insanity of eating too much is at the forefront of my mind. As I watch the television the advertiser's deception infuriates me. I think, we must, as mature adults, help future generations protect their minds from these evil manipulators that are out to make money from people buying their client's crap! Obviously not all advertising is this way, but a vast majority is nothing more than a form of brainwashing.

It is well documented that if we do not eat for hours or days, it gives our bodies a break from the busy work of digesting and a healing process quickly takes over. I am convinced that when people get admitted to the hospital, the simple act of not eating (IV drip) is a major contributor to why they sometimes feel better.

Fasting has long been known to be beneficial both mentally and physically so why don't we teach our children to skip a lunch from time to time? "Eat to keep that strength up" is instead rammed in young minds! Teachers, doctors and parents are all guilty. Eat, eat, these authority figures tell them! Perhaps we should re-think this or a new generation of food addicted people will be inevitable.

Think of the money you will save and the increase in the quality of living you will yield by eating less food. You will be able to watch your loved ones grow and be less of a burden on them as you age. You will not only be kinder to yourself but to Earth.

I have been blessed with many years of good health. I have eaten mostly a vegetarian diet and have benefited tremendously but I must eat less of everything. It is not worth it to overeat- simply not worth it. The small pleasures we gain by eating too much in the moment cause us too much pain and suffering in our futures.

I think back to the insanity of my workouts in my 30s. I was addicted to running, lifting, biking, swimming and this was all in the high altitude of Albuquerque New Mexico. I was 160 pounds with 6% body fat. Thinking back, I loved how I looked. I could eat what I wanted and not worry about weight gain. But I was eating way too much! I was addicted to the fact that I could eat whatever I wanted, if I kept the intense workouts up.

Finding the middle is the key! Workout out gently and eat gently!

I often think about how refreshing it would be to receive an invitation to a party that reads like this; "Come celebrate our 25th wedding anniversary with us! Fresh water, dancing, music and a variety of fresh fruits served. Organic wine and beer provided!" Why not, I ask? Would it kill us not to eat for a few hours and celebrate life without junk food that causes us so much pain and suffering?

Instead, we serve cake and ice cream to our kids and smile like it is so cute. Do we realize that these kids get a temporary "high" because they are consuming a drug (processed sugar)? We say, "A little is ok" but is it?

This is only day 3 and I feel more alive and my mind is full of energy. I can write easily.

I started this book last year but only lasted a couple of weeks as it was during the holidays and I just could not keep up with the pace of social eating and so called celebration. This time I know I will not fail. I recently watched the documentary Fat, Sick and Nearly Dead and it inspired me to write again.

Summary of food intake from day 3:

16 ounces of banana, strawberry and melon smoothie: 300 calories

16 ounces of kale, beat, apple, carrot and lemon juice: 300 calories

Large salad of mixed veggies: 350 calories

Total calories: 950

Exercise: 12-mile bike ride and some free weights.

Thoughts from my bike ride: I have been urinating more than usual and pooping more frequently.

DAY: 4

WEIGHT: 207
DATE: JULY 31, 2016

"To change a habit, make a conscious decision, then act the new behavior." Maxwell Maltz

I almost jumped out of bed this morning as my mind was racing with thoughts and my energy level is high.

So how does one accomplish a goal like this with his back against society's walls of compromise? I mean to say, with so many negative influences around you, that becomes a challenge. There is junk food available everywhere and negative people surround us like a bad cold.

My family and I moved to Plainfield Indiana in 2001 (1 month after 911). Prior to that move, we lived in Albuquerque since 1989. The adjustment was difficult, being vegetarians from sunny Albuquerque. However, we quickly made friends and adapted to this place we live to this day. People are solid and willing to lend a hand and I am appreciative of our close friends. Although, we have very few friends that are vegetarians, I can see we have been a positive influence on some of their dietary choices.

When I lived in New Mexico I was a television talk show host for a public show called "Ask the Vegetarian." This was not a ram it down your throat sort of show. It was more of a relaxed show that covered topics about the benefits of a vegetarian diet.

My good friend, Don Schrader was a local activist that influenced me to start the show and was a major influence in my life. To this day, Don is extremely active in the Albuquerque community with his message of simple living and eating a plant based diet. He lives on less than 10,000 a year and eats only a raw plant based diet. This guy is the real deal. We used to call him the Real Jesus as he was living what he preached.

In the must read book, Psycho-Cybernetics by Maxwell Maltz, Maltz thoroughly examines the correlation between how we perceive ourselves and self-esteem. In short, the physical and mental aspects of our existence are connected. So, I cannot help but think that many of us could benefit tremendously by eating less food in which would allow one to maintain a healthy weight. Thus, increasing self-esteems that would enrich lives in incredible ways.

I dream of socializing events that offer walks in the woods, great conversation and small amounts of healthy food.

Wouldn't it be nice, for a change, to just exist, rather than continually digging our own graves with our teeth? My point is, that it seems like most everything we do involves unhealthy foods.

I think of all the days I wasted eating too much food, along with the wasted money, not to mention compromising my self-image. Thus, comprising my life. A life of compromise is no way to live. The good news is it is not too late to change.

We have all eaten too much at dinner and spent the rest of the night in sweatpants, watching TV. This is stupid, isn't it? Reverse the situation, where you ate a nice small plate of nutritious food and you spent the rest of the evening outdoors, enjoying life as it was meant to be. Everyone at one point or another in their lives can relate to this.

My body is already reshaping itself and I can feel myself turning a corner. As the first few days of a fast are the toughest I see easier roads ahead. Which supports my theory that food, not drugs are our number 1 addiction. Drugs have a withdrawal time of about 3 days. Thus, similar withdrawal times seem to correlate both with food and drug addictions. However, food is a more accepted addiction in our society. This is because literally most all of us have been brainwashed since childhood with reward systems where food is the reward to satisfy our most primitive needs.

Thus, this sort of venture is a reshaping, a reprogramming and you will have to get over this hump of withdrawal to have success. In short, you will have to be strong. Yes, if you have thought by now, it would be easier to place yourself in an environment where you could have a gentle go of it. As an example, go to Hawaii for a month or a lake retreat.

However, as we all know, economics plays a role, as in my life, in many lives. So, work with what you have and do the best you can.

A vivid observation I keep having is what people eat and buy at the grocery store. The horrendous, overcooked, charred, processed food we consume, along with the sheer amount is at the forefront of one's mind when fasting. Going to a grocery store or restaurant takes on an entirely different experience. Your awareness is at its peak and you cannot help but feel, just by looking at others food choices that disease, depression and self-esteem issues, linger with the multitudes of people in this country.

Summary from day 4:

32 ounces of kale, carrot, apple, beet and ginger juice: 550 calories

1 large salad: 400 calories

Total calories: 1050

Exercise: Some free weights.

Thoughts from today: As I watched TV today, the evil advertiser's attempt to brainwash me into buying their client's poison. Arby's uses the guy with that "tough" voice to hustle their bacon, turkey, meat sandwich on to hard working people with loved ones expecting them to live a long life. But instead, the truth is, many people will age horrendously as a result of the shit they eat.

DAY: 5
WEIGHT: NO WEIGHT RECORDED
DATE: AUGUST 1, 2016

"Willpower isn't something that gets handed out to some and not to others. It is a skill you can develop through understanding and practice." Gillian Riley

It is only the 5th day and I am only down a few pounds, but my mind feels sharp and I have noticed my skin has cleared up from a long time mild eczema issue on my knee and shoulder.

This venture has not really been difficult with exception of a couple of hungry moments. I feel better but I realize this lifestyle choice needs to go on for a couple of months for me to get the full scope of it. I am keeping my emotions in check, not to go too high or too low.

When you are fully conscious of your food choices and the amounts you eat, you start to observe others around you. It is like being sober in a bar full of drunk people. People are constantly, unconsciously stuffing food into their mouths. Horrible foods, full of sugar, white flour and high in animal fat.

I am convinced this behavior is the path to least resistance. We simply do not realize that our food choices carry on from generation to generation.

It feels much better to just exist than to have useless conversation over high fat cinnamon rolls. Isn't this true? Try it sometime. Try being silent without a need for any stimulants.

My mind is exploding with thoughts of food abuse and its intimate connection to everything that we do, and it seems to get worst with age. Our youth do not seem to need so much food around them to socialize but the adults cannot seem to function without it.

Summary from day 5:

16 ounces of mixed vegetable juice: 300 calories

Large mixed salad: 400 calories

Small salad: 250 calories

Total calories: 950

Exercise: Rode my bike 12 miles and some free weights

Thoughts from my bike ride: I just kept telling myself I can do this, and I am well on my way. Not to ever quit!

DAY: 6

WEIGHT: 205
DATE: AUGUST 2, 2016

"Peoples love of sweets and guilty feelings about overindulgence are pretty universal." Will Cotton

I have never been a sweets person but from time to time I have been known to indulge, especially chocolate. However, this is not the case for most. Sweets are basically a slow death warrant that destroys our health. So why do we eat them? Because it is a reward system developed from an early age that has been planted in our subconscious minds. But we look at this behavior as "cute" and some almost have a sexual sort of relationship with sweets, as they make groaning noises as they stuff cake and cookies in their mouths. When we realize this is a drug, not food, we might stop to act so silly.

Maintaining this lifestyle choice is especially difficult in Indiana. This is due to the influences around one and the scarcity of healthier food choices.

I believe one takes on her environment. The food choices, the weather, the habits, customs, all of it. Thus, it is important if you desire a healthy life, as does everyone, that you place yourself around like minded people. Otherwise, it is a harder climb up that mountain to enlightenment. Although, it is still very possible to achieve, you will just have to try harder.

Food takes on an entirely new meaning when you are on a fast. Potato chips look and smell like poison and fresh tomatoes jump out at you and explode with flavor. Awareness soars to new heights. My body feels like its healing, yet I have no known health issues other than carrying around a few extra pounds. I am excited for this new life, a life committed to being as good as I can be. I press on.

Summary from day 6:

32 ounces of carrot, beat and tomato juice: 550 calories

Large salad: 400 calories

Total calories: 900

Exercise: 13-mile bike ride

Thoughts from my bike ride: I am dreaming of the future and it is bright.

DAY: 7
WEIGHT: 204
DATE: AUGUST 3, 2016

"You are a product of your environment. So choose the environment that will best develop you toward your objective. Analyze your life in terms of its environment. Are the things around you helping you toward success - or are they holding you back?" W. Clement Stone

Since youth we have all heard the saying, "you are a product of your environment". However, as we grow older, we seem to melt into the same routines and our influences engulf us. As we age it becomes more difficult to break out of that routine. Thus, when it comes to living a life to the fullest, a whole food- plant based diet becomes distant. Our doctors tell us to cut back on fatty foods and to lose a few pounds, but they placate to us by saying that fasting and taking extreme measures is unrealistic. But is it? I think not! I think, again, we take a path to least resistance and we simply settle for mediocrity.

Today, I felt like my colon cleaned out. To put it mildly, I shit 5 times and felt like I lost 5 pounds of "gunk" from my body. I feel good today. I am not hungry, other than late night, but a salad will get me through. My appreciation level for food cannot be described. One must fast, to fully understand.

At no other time in the history of society has it been so crucial to have common sense-intuition to survive this monster plethora of advertisers we have bombarding us to eat more. They show you happy people eating junk food on TV, but the reality is that most of it is poison. Wendy's, Kellogg's and Hershey, to name a few, have but one goal; to push their shit on you for more profit.

It seems that most of us would love to be able to eat what we want and as much as we want, while losing or maintaining our weight. This is fundamentally wrong because ideal weight is not just how you look but how your body is functioning inside. If we have such thinking, we are only focusing on the visual aspects of our being and not the broader picture of food addiction.

Could we feed the entire world if all of us ate significantly less and would health care cost be cut in half? One does not need to dig very deep to find this to be true.

Summary from day 7:

Large mixed salad: 350 calories

16 ounces of tomato and cucumber juice: 300 calories

16 ounces of banana, honey dew, and strawberry smoothie: 300 calories

Total calories: 900

Exercise: None

Thoughts from today: The benefits of eating less are not only beneficial to ourselves but to the planet as well. Additionally, a conscious choice to eat less teaches discipline and your appreciation for food will be increased dramatically. Also, it can be fun and challenging.

DAY: 8

WEIGHT: 202
DATE: AUGUST 4, 2016

"Running alone is the toughest. You get to the point where you have to keep pushing yourself." Walter Payton

I have not told many that I am writing this journal, so my only support system is myself. I feel this is especially tough to accomplish but the above quote helps me push on alone!

I find it ironic that many seem more interested in their lawns than their health.

We can clearly see our lawns and immediately see results, whether we care for it or neglect it. But with our bodies, we cannot see what is going on inside. Thus, what we do not see, we do not worry about. It appears we only take charge of our bodies when a doctor tells us to and many times that is too late.

It is fascinating to me that we put our immediate gratification of meat and junk foods ahead of our long-term futures. We carefully invest in retirement funds but carelessly pollute our bodies.

Charles Caprarella

Summary from day 8:

16 ounces of tomato and green pepper juice: 300 calories

16 ounces of green apple, cucumber, cabbage and lemon juice: 300 calories

Large salad: 350

Total calories: 950

Exercise: 13-mile bike ride and some free weights

Thoughts from my bike ride: I will face much criticism for this little book. Many will say I am nuts or that I have an eating disorder. I will assure them that this is not the case. This is a conscious choice, and I am facing the reality of widespread food addiction in our society that contributes greatly to too much pain and suffering. Too much!

DAY: 9
WEIGHT: 202
DATE: AUGUST 5, 2016

"No one saves us but ourselves. No one can and no one may. We ourselves must walk the path." Buddha

I woke up feeling energetic, but I had a harder time sleeping than usual. My mind is racing with good thoughts and I am feeling like age healing is taking place within my body and mind. Its only day 9.

Many of us working adults work or have worked inside a building were people sit most of the day and glare into a computer screen. Then we come home, sit more and watch that death box, called a TV. I am not saying I have not watched my share of television or I am better than anyone else, but it is nevertheless a death box, metaphorically speaking.

My point is that if we seek the good life we need to lobby at our jobs. Request workout rooms and PTO that encourages good health and a positive working environment. To elaborate, I do not mean walks around the building and yogurt and salad for lunch 3 days a week. I am talking about going entire weeks without any cooked food, charred animal flesh or processed foods. This is an all-out commitment to yourself, the planet, and world hunger. Sometimes compromise and moderation can be weak terms.

I can assure you this. If you brought a vegetable juicer into the work break room and juiced for 2 weeks straight, others would follow by your example. Putting micronutrient food in your body and saying no to junk foods takes serious work and humility.

What is a comfort food anyway? I believe it is food that satisfies the part of the brain that gives us instant satisfaction. Our minds are a result of years of impressions being seen on the television and what society has taught us.

I have been a vegetarian for many years and as a result have been insulted and poked fun of. We get questions like, "how do you get your protein" and "what do you eat at thanksgiving." This just comes with the territory and it is a form of deflection and insecurities from meat eaters.

It is true if everyone started to count calories, it would have a profound economic impact, but we would have a healthier world where food was honored more than abused. Isn't it worth it?

Summary from day 9:

16 ounces of carrot, green apple and lemon juice. 300 calories

16 ounces of banana, strawberry and pineapple smoothie. 300 calories

Large salad: 300

3 lite beers: 350

Soy based foods when I got home from a concert: 600 calories

Total calories: 1850

Exercise: 12-mile bike ride

Thoughts from my bike ride: Again, it is crucial we learn to live on less food, less calories and transform to foods packed with micronutrients. If we humans do not stop eating so much, we will not only destroy ourselves, but we destroy future generation's ability to survive. I once read somewhere that if everyone just fasted for one day a week that we would stop world hunger in its tracks. Maybe that is a bit outrageous, but I do not think it is too far off.

DAY: 10
WEIGHT: 202
DATE: AUGUST 6, 2016

"The best preparation for tomorrow is doing your best today."
H. Jackson Brown, Jr.

Yesterday was my first "walk off path" but today I am back on course.

It is important to stock your home with good foods so that when you do get weak, and you will from time to time, you can at least "pig out" on somewhat healthier foods. But keeping high fat processed foods around is not a good move. So why do people buy these items? Because it is easy, and one cannot escape a lifetime of an early childhood food reward system unless one realizes that their number one addiction in their lives is food and those choices can contribute to life or death.

My goal is not to placate to you but to make you think. Thinking, even in disagreement, causes change. If you want to flip your life around, turn back father time, feel 25 again, then massive change will be required.

I can only write so much as each day passes but I feel as though the writing is keeping me motivated. No matter what diet one adopts, I think that starting a journal would be greatly beneficial as it keeps one accountable.

It is getting easier to say no to food as my mind is being re-conditioned. By keeping this journal, I feel as though I am accountable to succeed in this quest in which feels so right.

Centering our activities on food is truly the path to least resistance and the path to destroying our health, limiting our ability to live life to the fullest. Again, I expect to be criticized but radical moves bring resistance. My long-term hope is that others will start to follow, by the end of this journey.

Summary from day 10:

16 ounces of carrot, green apple and cabbage juice: 300

Large salad (with seeds): 450 calories

Some almonds: 250 calories

Total calories: 1000

Thoughts from my bike ride: I totally blew it last night but today I went back on track.

DAY: 11
WEIGHT: 201
DATE: AUGUST 7, 2016

"Oh, pity the poor glutton
Whose troubles all begin
In struggling on and on to turn
What's out into what's in." Walter de la Ma

I am now 11 days in, and it feels longer, as if this is the way I have always eaten. It is amazing to me how resilient our bodies are, its ability to heal and correct itself.

Much of my life, I have been astonished by junk food that is masked as "good cheer", yet many people suffer with depression, bloated stomachs, sickness, lack of energy and trips to the emergency room. No doubt these food choices we have adopted in America is contributing greatly to our demise in countless ways.

It is well documented that restricting calorie intake is beneficial to longevity and quality of life. Equally important is that eating micronutrient rich foods enrich our cells. Also, for your best bang for your buck, if you eliminate all animal foods from your diet, you will thrive. Yes, as you may be thinking, this can be an extreme change for most people, yet a change that will add years of quality living to your life.

So called professionals could argue that this diet choice is too extreme, however, on the other hand, equally as many professionals would agree with me. At the end of the day, it is obviously your choice what to eat but one must feel lucky to have that choice. Imagine living in many areas of the world, still, were that luxury to choose is simply unavailable. We are lucky!

Summary from day 11:

16 ounces of banana and strawberry smoothie: 300 calories

16 ounces of cucumber, green apple and lemon juice: 300 calories

Large salad: 350 calories

Total calories: 950

Exercise: 11-mile bike ride

Thoughts from my bike ride: I feel hopeful today.

DAY: 12

WEIGHT: 201
DATE: AUGUST 8, 2016

"If we do not voluntarily bring population growth under control in the next one or two decades, then nature will do it for us in the most brutal way, whether we like it or not." Henry W. Kendall

Population growth is out of control with an increase of over 6 billion people in the last 100 years. This along with overeating could create a starving world soon. Thus- food conservation and population control are large factors for the future of the planet. Eating less will greatly contribute to this fact, as well as eating lower on the food chain. In the book Diet for a Small Planet by Frances Moore Lappé, he explains in detail the devastating impact that animal foods have on our environment. I highly recommend reading this book.

It is impossible to live cruelty free, as it has been proven in science that all living things, plant or animal, feel pain to an extent. However, to live on a plant based diet not only makes common sense but it is a way of not contributing to the inhumane treatment of animals, not to mention the devastating impact that flesh consumption has on the echo system. Furthermore, we are herbivores by nature, not carnivores. People will argue this point but it is quite obvious that if we humans were really meat eaters, per say, then why in the hell do we need to cook food? Why doesn't a baby look at a chicken and want to bite its head off?

My body feels somewhat lighter today, but I do not expect to feel a significant difference until I am well below 200 pounds. At my height of 5'10" my ideal body weight is 160 to 170.

My juicer unexpectedly died today so I MUST go get a new one. This was a Hamilton Beach Model, so I guess I will not buy that one again. I could tell the motor was slowly going but this is bummer to have to buy a new one already. I shopped around and bought a Black and Decker for $34.95. It works well but you must chop things up because the feeder is smaller. However, it seems as though that process puts less strain on the motor. This is a good buy and does the job for 1 person at a time, but it takes a little longer to juice.

I am pooping 3 times a day on a regular basis now and I must say, it feels as though I am taking in a lot of quality food in and a good amount of toxins-waste is going out.

Summary from day 12:

16 ounces of carrot, apple, ginger and beat juice: 300 calories

16 ounces of banana and strawberry smoothie: 300 calories

Small salad: 200 calories

Baked potato: 200 calories

Total calories: 1000

Exercise: None

Thoughts from today: I cheated some today, but life goes on.

DAY: 13
WEIGHT: 199
DATE: AUGUST 9, 2016

"Without deviation from the norm, progress is not possible."
Frank Zappa

"Every individual is, in a way, a combination of Life and Death. Everything you do contributes to either of these two aspects. So when you eat, a simple thought, will this contribute to life or death, should be practiced." *Sadhguru*

Today I am under 200 pounds. As a result, I am anxious to continue and my confidence is soaring!

I love the above quote. Should I eat steak or salad? Steak is death in more ways than one. It represents a dead tortured cow that will be digested by your body and your body will make deposits of that throughout. Salad is alive with nutrients and thus the opposite will occur. A box of crackers will not do anything much but satisfy your taste buds and so on and so forth. So, each time we eat, it is either a deposit or a withdrawal.

Charles Caprarella

In the book, Psycho-Cybernetics by Maxwell Maltz, he brings the subject of self-esteem to the forefront and fluctuating weight certainly is a major contributor to low self-esteem. When we are happy with ourselves, we tend to have better relationships and live more positive lives. This is what we all want, isn't it?

I went shopping at Trader Joes today and I must say they offer healthier choices for a fair price. It is refreshing to shop amongst other healthy minded people, and it is nice to see businesses like that flourishing. Unfortunately, the traditional grocery stores are terribly busy too.

Have you ever been in line at the grocery store and looked at other people's carts in line? For me, I do this frequently and it is disheartening to see the crap that many people buy for themselves and their families.

It is not that we lack the knowledge as to why we eat too much of the bad things but it's the fact that we have become a lazy society that's allured by the ease and convenience of quick fix foods. The path to least resistants' is an easy path to take. You can easily break this habit, but it won't be easy.

The McDonald's drive-thru line is long on a consistent basis as people rush around and ram food down their throats. It is a quick fix and their commercial from the night before is freshly imbedded in the mind.

Summary from day 13:

16 ounces of cucumber, kale, carrot and apple juice: 300 calories

2 ounces of raw almonds: 400 calories

Large salad: 350 calories

Totals calories: 1050

Exercise: 12-mile bike ride

Thoughts from my bike ride: I did not drink as much juice today because I just didn't feel like cleaning up today as I was anticipating visiting my friend Eric in the hospital who is terminally ill with cancer. This guy, my buddy, is a 44-year-old warrior and one would be hard pressed to find someone nicer.

Eric has lived a life of eating bad foods and was a heavy smoker. Undoubtedly, if he could turn back time, he would have changed his ways. I am sad, to an unspeakable extent.

It was difficult to visit him in the hospital. I sat as he quivered in pain. He could barely sit up and consume some comfort foods. This was pink lemonade, ice cream and a snickers bar. These death items are masked pretty with packaging and advertising and even have a hold on someone in their last days. Shame on the hospital to offer these items. Shame on the doctors and nurses who do not protest these items. It was sheer agony to watch.

DAY: 14
WEIGHT: 199
DATE: AUGUST 10, 2016

"Life is too short to waste any amount of time on wondering what other people think about you. In the first place, if they had better things going on in their lives, they wouldn't have the time to sit around and talk about you. What's important to me is not others' opinions of me, but what's important to me is my opinion of myself." C. Joy Bell

I have only told a few people about this journal, my attempt to fast, lose a lot of weight and adopt a diet only consisting of plant based foods. I have gotten some laughs, rolling of the eyes but I am fortunate to have great support from many. Interestingly, much of the support is coming from the young instead of middle aged adults that seem to be set in their ways.

Like many Americans, many of those negative people are very sickly. They take pills for high blood pressure and diabetes, have already had many surgeries, suffer from endless ailments and are overall lethargic and tired.

But they are so brainwashed by the typical American doctor that they think there is extraordinarily little correlation between what you eat and how you feel. Most chalk it up to genetics or "when it's your time it's your time." For a thinker, like myself and you, this sort of attitude is incomprehensible.

Some have changed their ways that I have known but many just think I'm a whacko and that's the way it is. I avoid most debates these days because honestly, I would not have many friends if I frankly spoke my mind.

My friend Eric, father of 2, is a hardworking great guy and loving husband. He was diagnosed with 4th stage lung cancer on January 15, 2016 at 44 years old. At the time, I urged him to take the holistic route instead of the so called "medical cure."

Now 7 months later he has weeks to live. The chemo, "treatments" and radiation cost hundreds of thousands of dollars and assuredly helped pay some big doctor salaries and overpaid hospital administrator's but did little for Eric.

The food you eat becomes you. Your body regenerates itself with the food so every time you eat something, if its healthy food or junk food, it becomes part of who you are. So why not make good choices?

In life we need to be our own best doctors. At no other time in the history of the world have we had the ability to be on a similar level with intellectuals that were once only part of the formally educated group. This is due to technology. We can use Google and YouTube for just about any subject. Yes, you cannot believe everything you read but your common sense can usually help you make choices between fact and fiction.

Summary from day 14:

32 ounces of carrot, beat, green apple, tomato and cucumber juice. 500 calories

Large salad: 500 calories

1 ounce of raw almonds: 200 calories

Total calories: 1200

Exercise: None

Thoughts from today: This new juicer does the job. It's much smaller so you have to prep vegetables better, but the yield is good and it's quieter and self-contained. At $34.95, I am happy.

I went to the hospital to visit Eric tonight. My daughter, Sydney, Eric's son Tyler, Eric's father Phil and Mother Liz were in the room. Laughter, reflection and conversation filled the air. Then, without warning, like a bulldozer, Dr. X walks in and gives us a quick warning. "Are you all family" he asked? I pause; however, Eric says, "Of course." Like a bat out of hell, the doctor proceeds to say this. "Eric I am going to level with you…. you will die from this cancer and there is NO cure! But maybe we can buy you some time! Eric quivered in shock- his eyes exploding open, as tears shed. "We are talking a year or two," Says Eric, trying to put a few words together. "No no no, you don't have that kind of time," says doc in his Indian accent. "But despite what your other doctor said (no point in trying another round of chemo), you are young and perhaps there is an outside chance we can put "this thing" in remission and buy you a few months. So, it is something to think about.

There is nobody to blame here, these things can happen to anyone despite what they eat. But one cannot help but think of the countless times this very scenario could have been avoided by dietary choices. This is not my opinion. It is well documented that people and cultures that consume foods lower on the food chain, live longer and with dramatically less illness.

DAY: 15
WEIGHT: 198
DATE: AUGUST 11, 2016

"Let's be clear. The planet is not in jeopardy. We are in jeopardy. We haven't got the power to destroy the planet - or to save it. But we might have the power to save ourselves." Michael Crichton, Jurassic Park

The way we eat and its impact on the planet is widely known. It has been shown that the greatest negative impact on Earth is meat production and consumption. The meat and dairy industries spend billions of dollars making sure our teachers, parents and doctors are well informed to help brainwash our youth. Fact is that their products contribute greatly to the destruction of the planet and human health. Thus, it would behoove us to cut back on the consumption of meat and dairy products.

As I suspected it is getting easier to be fully conscious of the amount of food, I am eating each day. Our subconscious mind does more work than we know. If we feed it well, we get positive results. But the subconscious does not distinguish between good and bad, it just is. So, considering the fact that we are brainwashed from birth to associate food with just about everything, it won't be an easy task to change your habits.

Summary from day 15:

16 ounces of carrot, cucumber, beets and apple juice: 300 calories

16 ounce banana and blueberries smoothie: 300c calories

Vegetable soup: 250 calories

1 large salad: 400 calories

Totals calories: 1250

Exercise: 12 mile bike ride. 40 push-ups, 30 sit-ups.

Thoughts from my bike ride: We live in an enlightened age of human existence, thanks to technology. It is so easy to look things up and I do believe doctors get annoyed by the "know it all" but it is our bodies so we need to take control and be our own best doctors.

DAY: 16
WEIGHT: 197
DATE: AUGUST 12, 2016

"Patience is not simply the ability to wait - it's how we behave while we're waiting." *Joyce Meyer*

There is no doubt in my mind that where you live contributes greatly to your eating habits. The food choices in the Midwest, being a meat and potatoes place, are simply not as good as some other more progressive areas but then again, perhaps I would not have come to this point without the experience.

I think we tend to take on the characteristics of our environment so placing yourself in a proper proximity will only benefit you. If you want to be an actor, move to Hollywood. If you want to be a surfer, move to Hawaii. You know what I mean?

I have no weight loss to report today but I am feeling lighter in my mind and good about the near future. I can feel the healing process taking place as my body thanks me every day for not making it work so hard to eliminate excessive food from my body.

My venture is a challenge, as the dead of summer offers beer and cheer. The advertisers of processed foods and booze trick us well to believe that our path to enlightenment is through their clients.

When I was a child, I would gaze at so called authority figures when they would bellow stupid words like, "Eat your meat" and "drink your milk for strong bones." I somehow knew it was all a pack of lies and went on to enjoy health and fitness without hardly consuming any meat or milk. I maintained muscle and weight and no broken bones. I was active and excelled at sports.

As I was cleaning the kitchen today (from my daughters' tofu-pasta-vegetable casserole), I was reflecting on how much money is wasted on food. Many recipes urge us to cook monstrously complicated dishes that require, eggs, cheese, creams and animal flesh. It is like preparing a small slice of death. If you really examine many recipes posted on social media and cookbooks, you will find this to be true. Wouldn't it be a better world if we ate simpler, using all natural whole food ingredients?

Although a seemingly extreme statement, our refrigerators are good for nothing but preserving dying foods and should eventually be eliminated from your kitchen for maximum health benefits. Not to mention refrigeration has a negative impact on mother earth. So why not keep whole foods in a cool place and eliminate that refrigerator?

Many will have good arguments about this sensitive subject but as for me, my body and health are all I really must call home so being selfish for the betterment of it is something I am willing to live with. I for one, without family votes, would not own a refrigerator.

It is just something to think about. My attempt here is not to sound superior to anyone but just to get you thinking. To reiterate, our food choices do not make us better or worse than the next person.

To expand, I am not against technology. I just think we need to be extremely selfish when it comes to our bodies and health and do what is best for it. Without question, as we each become healthier, collectively, society benefits. Health care cost would plummet and the massive budgets and debt for health care would be at least cut in half. The world would be a better place, isn't it so?

Today the weather forecast is brutally hot and humid, but it appears that cooler days are ahead. Cooler weather is nice for bike rides and gives me an overall feeling of energy and vitality. Fall in Indiana, from about mid-August to mid-November is wonderful, offering pleasant days and cooler nights. However, the rest of the months are mostly harsh.

Summary from day 16:

16 ounce banana, honey dew, blueberries and ice smoothie: 300

1 large plate of steamed broccoli: 300

2 ounces of cashews: 400

Totals calories: 1000

Exercise: 12 mile bike ride. 45 push-ups. 45 sit-ups.

Thoughts from my bike ride: Despite the 90 degree heat and humidity, my bike ride today was especially easy.

DAY: 17
WEIGHT: 196
DATE: AUGUST 13, 2016

"On the Continent people have good food; in England people have good table manners." George Mikes

Tonight, will be challenging. I am to attend a get together with friends and the closest thing to healthy food will be cream based dishes with some vegetables added. The dishes will be presented well in expensive cookware. Of course, meat dishes will be readily available. This is meat and potatoes USA. This is not always the case, but Indiana is a little behind when it comes to being health conscious.

Quickly, within 10 minutes after we arrived, they gathered like hungry cats, around the kitchen counter and stuffed piles of pork shoulder in their mouths. I could almost visualize the flesh working its way around their body's as their body worked desperately to process this highly toxic, burnt animal remain. Washing it down with beer.

It is well known that our body cannot metabolize alcohols well, so when you combine alcohol with animal flesh the body puts alcohol as its number one priority to quickly eliminate alcohol from your body. It is called metabolic priority. As a result, the flesh rots as it waits its turn to be distributed to vital organs and cells. Some of the flesh gets distributed to build muscle and feed the cells but much of it gets stored in organs and arterial walls. This is a deadly combination, but this scenario (mixing meat and alcohol) takes place on a monumental level, every day, in the millions. It is no wonder our hospitals are packed, and the drug companies laugh all the way to the bank.

The evil advertisers and animal food companies howl at the moon, with profits in the trillions, as you help their evil empires plot destruction with your consumptions.

They are solid people at this get together, hardworking, honest and proud. So, it is difficult to observe their slow demise and their withering of health right before my eyes. I say nothing though. The words I would say would be met with harsh criticism, as in the past, and would have done more damage than good. I just sit and placate for the moment and think that hopefully, by writing these words, I can somehow make a difference soon.

Foods appearance seems to be more important than the actual food itself. We add useless ingredients that ruin the food as it was intended to be eaten. Heavy cheeses and cream sauces loaded with saturated fat and cholesterol are added to mask the so called blandness of the whole foods.

Summary from day 17:

16 ounce carrot, cucumber, tomato, beet and apple juice: 300

1 large salad: 300

A variety of vegetables and fresh salsa: 300

Some pasta salad: 150

Totals calories: 1050

Exercise: 10 mile bike ride. 40 push-ups. 40 sit-ups.

Thoughts from my bike ride: This was a difficult day because of this party I went to but at least it gave me something good to write about. I gave in to a few more calories than I thought I would be oh well.

DAY: 18

WEIGHT: 196
DATE: AUGUST 14, 2016

"Exercise to stimulate, not to annihilate. The world wasn't formed in a day, and neither were we. Set small goals and build upon them." Lee Haney

My goal with exercise is to not depend on it. But the above quote hits home for me. I have always been an exerciser but at times I was obsessed with it and enjoyed the fact that I could eat what I wanted. However, one must know that the exterior person is not the interior person. As an example, a great looking body does not mean it is a healthy or happy body. Our accumulation of food is the truth of the matter and is a deposit or withdrawal every time we choose what we eat.

No loss on the scale today but more and more I am thinking less about weight loss as I know this sort of commitment brings a pleasant weight and my body, a marvelous machine, takes care of everything for me. All I must do is feed it correctly. Additionally, everyone has a different body style and goal so in a sense, appearance is overrated but we all react the same biologically. Thus, the way you feel is more important. The goal should be to get off of medications, if possible, and heal yourself from high-blood pressure and many other pill fed ailments you may have.

I am feeling good about myself. The flow and ease of it gets more normal each day.

GMO foods are a controversial topic today and I cannot help but think that the amounts of food we consume contribute greatly to this subject because most of us eat too much. I think if we all cut our food consumption in half that world hunger would be aided greatly.

Health care would be cut considerably. We always say, "Our health is more important than money, don't we?" We must start somewhere if we expect change and this change will come with a price.

Summary from day 18:

16 ounce carrot, beat and tomato juice: 300

Large salad: 350

Totals calories: 650

Exercise: 12 mile bike ride. 50 push-ups. 50 sit-ups.

Thoughts from my bike ride:

Let us be honest, brutally honest, food addiction in this country is a leach on our souls and causing horrendous amounts of undue suffering, rapid aging and there is no end in sight. But it is easily curable, today! Just make the right decisions as to what you put in your mouth. It is that easy!

DAY: 19

WEIGHT: 195
DATE: AUGUST 15, 2016

"Everybody looks at their poop." Oprah Winfrey

I heard a long time ago that it is not what you eat but what you shit. So, I inquired more about this subject and it makes perfect sense. What comes out of your body is just as important as what goes in. One does not need to research long to realize this truth. If you are shitting well, you are usually well.

You hear a lot about protein in the diet but when you investigate further one finds that it is mostly propaganda and a heavily funded myth by the meat and dairy industry. Fact is, and this is the short version, that a diet consisting of more than 30% protein creates havoc on your body and animal protein is a toxic poison!

I have taken a few supplements over the years but let us face it, this stuff doesn't work. The protein supplement business is a 2.7 billion a year industry and you can find as many articles showing the benefits as you can the negative. But what do you do? How do you choose? Do what you want but I choose to use my common sense here? You?

My body is 17 pounds lighter since I started this, and I must admit I don't feel that much thinner but my clothes are fitting a little better and people are commenting that I look slimmer. I think in another 10 pounds or so things will start to rapidly progress. I can feel my body changing for the better.

Each day, I feel more toxins are being flushed as I continue this quest.

Charles Caprarella

Summary from day 19:

16 ounce banana and strawberry smoothie: 300

Large salad: 400

20 ounces of kale, carrot, ginger and apple juice: 400

Totals calories: 1100

Exercise: Biked 13 miles. 75 push-ups. 50 sit ups.

Thoughts from my bike ride: Keep pushing!

DAY: 20

WEIGHT: 194
DATE: AUGUST 16, 2016

"The food we eat goes beyond its macronutrients of carbohydrates, fat and protein. It's information. It interacts with and instructs our genome with every mouthful, changing genetic expression."
David Perlmutter

We are truly what we eat. For me, at day 20 on this modified juice fast, my mind is blowing open, my body is shedding pounds and strangely, I feel closer to oneness than ever. It is difficult for me to think that the food we eat does not shape us in ways we cannot see or comprehend.

Spiritually speaking let us think for a minute. When one consumes a cow that has been tortured, mutilated and caged for its entire life, isn't it possible that our souls, spirit, the unseen, could be intertwined with that tormented animal?

Today I feel like I have turned a corner. I do not feel nearly as hungry and I get full easy. It's obvious my stomach is shrinking, and my subconscious mind is feeding my conscious mind better choices.

Summary from day 20:

16 ounces of romaine lettuce, ginger, tomato and beet juice: 300

16 ounces of ginger, carrot, cucumber and celery juice: 300

Huge salad: 500

Totals calories: 1100

Exercise: 15 mile bike ride. 50 push-ups.

Thoughts from my bike ride: I just enjoyed nature and did not think about anything.

DAY: 21
WEIGHT: 194
DATE: AUGUST 17, 2016

"No one saves us but ourselves. No one can and no one may. We ourselves must walk the path." Buddha

This life can offer so many great opportunities when we make the right choices and choose our own path. For me, I frequently sit in silence, dream and read many things about many different subjects. My mother used to tell me we come in alone and leave alone. That is harsh but I think she meant it in a broader sense. To question authority!

Knowledge has never been so readily available today because of the internet so take advantage of that and question everything along the way.

Last night I went to visit Eric at Hendricks County Hospital. Watching someone pass on makes one realize how alive we really are. Witnessing someone die from cancer makes one think about lifestyle choices and its correlation to this nightmare of a disease.

Of course, not all cancers are caused by lifestyle, but I have read a multitude of studies that indicate that as much as 70% of all illness is self-inflicted by dietary and lifestyle choices. It makes sense to think that choosing to eat mostly a plant based diet would greatly reduce the odds of getting cancer.

The visit was nice but heart wrenching!

To take on this task to write this book was a decision I made by myself. I feel that paths are personal and sometimes you just need to walk them without advice or opinions. Just do it, as they say. I walk alone but there are many like me!

My weight is the same today and I feel well. My body appears to be getting tighter and my energy is up. It is a great feeling to wake up a little hungry and my clothes are looser.

I read an article that said as much as 80% of all soy in the USA is now GMO (genetically modified). I am making sure to read labels. I am not qualified to speak in detail on GMO foods, but it seems to make sense to stay away as much as possible.

On one hand I can see the need for GMOs as our population base in the world continues to grow but if I have a choice, ill choose non GMO. Our population has increased about six billion in the last 100 years. I have read estimates that if population growth continues that as much as a third of the human population will be starving in 50 years. Another reason to eat less.

Summary from day 21:

28 ounce ginger, apple, lime, carrot, celery and beet juice: 450

Peas and corn: 200

Vegetable fajita: 500

Total calories: 1150

Exercise: 15 mile bike ride. 50 sit-ups. 60 push-ups.

Thoughts from my bike ride: Why do we get fat in America as we age and why is it widely accepted? I feel that it is because we choose to, we simply choose. We choose to accept this as fact- since it's easy to eat, it's easy to sit and it's easy to not be creative in our planning when it comes to activities revolving around food. Most everything revolves around food. We exercise hours upon hours just so we can eat what we want. Pure insanity.

DAY: 22

WEIGHT: 194
DATE: AUGUST 18, 2016

"You have to keep pushing toward those dreams no matter what setbacks happen." Anthony Hamilton

This will be a challenging week because today I am helping my son relocate to the Denver area. We will be driving 17 hours by car, packed with personal belongings. I froze 32 ounces of vegetable juice for the ride and am bringing some raw almonds.

I know I will not be able to exercise today but I aim to do 75 or more pushups to keep my blood flowing and hopefully I can get through this trip without going off track too much but traveling will not be easy. When I get to Denver, I aim to look for some juice bars.

It is interesting to me that we have this "skinny" is not healthy attitude as we hear frequently the statement, "I don't feel comfortable at that weight". This to me is just an excuse to settle and continue our love affair with food. Also, we vegetarians hear the statement, "I could never give up meat or cheese." Personally, my mind does not work that way and I am not a never say never person. Quit or compromise is not in my DNA. Sadly, many are forced to change their eating habits when it is almost too late. If they hear it from a doctor after a heart attack its ok but they refuse to use their common sense. As an example: a woman has her first heart attack at 45 and now she is eating more salad and less meat and dairy. Why wait for the inevitable to happen?

I am not saying that one is 100% safe from heart disease if they rid themselves of all animal foods, but statistics show that their chances will be dramatically reduced by choosing to eat a plant based diet. It is a challenge, yes, but it is not exceedingly difficult in this world of abundant food choices.

Imagine a world were at birthday parties and weddings, healthy food is offered and that is the norm? Do you think that would be a better or worst world- is an honest question to ask yourself? Again, it would have a major impact on the economy as fast food restaurants would suffer, cake makers will have to get creative. Some hospitals would go out of business.

We arrived in a small town in Kansas, 3 hours from our destination and I did well. We stopped at a Chinese restaurant and I had steamed vegetables and rice but other than that I just had almonds and 32 ounces of juice.

Summary from day 22:

32 ounces of vegetable juice (mixed): 400

Almonds: 450

Steamed vegetables and rice: 400

Total calories: 1250

Exercise: 75 push-ups

Thoughts from today: Driving 17 hours in a car made my brain weary and all I was thinking of was a nice bed.

DAY: 23
WEIGHT: DID NOT WEIGH IN
DATE: AUGUST 19, 2016

"Never give up on something that you can't go a day without thinking about." Winston Churchill

Keeping this journal is imperative for I have been brainwashed since birth, to associate many activities with food. It is an everyday reminder.

We arrived in Golden Colorado after getting a good night sleep in a small hotel in Western Kansas. What a gorgeous area- wow! It was great traveling with my son Alec. We had in depth conversations about many subjects.

This lifestyle I suggest could be of major shock to many but to me it makes perfect sense. When you compare this lifestyle to getting your chest cut open or chemotherapy treatment, any sane person would choose it. But that is basically the choice we have. Facts are facts and the fact is, if you gorge on an animal food, your chances of heart disease and cancer get drastically increased.

Summary from day 23:

Massive salad and some pizza crust: 500

32 ounces of juice at a juice bar: 400

Miscellaneous raw foods: 400

Totals: 1300

Exercise: 50 push-ups

Thoughts of the day: I don't have a scale, so I won't weigh myself until I get back to Indiana.

DAY: 24

WEIGHT: DID NOT WEIGH IN
DATE: AUGUST 20, 2016

"Some days it is a heroic act just to refuse the paralysis of fear and straighten up and step into another day." Edward Albert

This is my second day in Colorado. We aim to run around all day, getting my sons new house set up and a variety of other chores.

As I observe Denver and the surrounding areas, I was surprised to see so many food chains, however, there are healthier choices than the Midwest has to offer. I could not help but think how we have become a society of chain restaurants and how are decisions where to eat are largely based on the impressions from advertisers we see on television. This coupled with convenience and branding is a money maker for them!

Summary from day 24:

32 ounces of juice from a juice bar: 450

Large salad and a variety of fresh vegetables and fruits: 600

Total calories: 1050

Exercise: 12 mile bike ride in Golden Colorado.

Thoughts from my bike ride: Wow this place is wonderful. Bike paths everywhere. I could get used to this.

DAY: 25
WEIGHT: DID NOT WEIGH IN
DATE: AUGUST 21, 2016

"Nothing will benefit human health and increase chances for survival of life on Earth as much as the evolution to a vegetarian diet. "Albert Einstein

At my age, 53, you hear so much from people about their variety of illnesses, that you cannot help but cringe at what they eat, and the amount they eat.

I myself have been a vegetarian for many years but certainly have cheated from time to time but for argument sake, 80% of the time I have eaten no animal based foods. As a result, I have enjoyed minimal health problems and not one night in the hospital. My vital signs or solid and I can still enjoy many activities as I did in my youth. Yes, I am slower but still capable of playing catch with my kids, swimming, bike rides, walking and hiking.

I only mention these things to show that even though I have battled with weight fluctuations I have enjoyed good health from mostly eating plants. In short, studies show, a chubby

Charles Caprarella

vegetarian is healthier than a skinny meat eater. There are too many studies to mention and it is a google search away.

Its day 25 and I am growing fully aware of everything around me. My mind is starting to explode with reality as I am fully focused on food and its relationship to our lives.

I feel good about myself and feel that I am making terrific progress, both mentally and physically. I look forward each day to writing down my progress and thoughts. I am starting to roll, and it is surprisingly easy.

Summary from day 25:

30 ounces of carrot, apple and ginger juice: 400

Popcorn: 300

Veggie rice: 400

Totals calories: 1100

Exercise: 15 miles of bike riding in the foothills of Golden. I need oxygen!

Thoughts from my bike ride: I could get used to riding in this place. The hills are challenging and feels great on my lungs and body.

DAY: 26

WEIGHT: DID NOT WEIGH IN
DATE: AUGUST 22, 2016

"You know that a majority of the medical costs that are bankrupting families, companies, and nations could be eliminated with better nutrition." John Robbins, Voices of the Food Revolution: You Can Heal Your Body and Your World—With Food!

It is so lovely when hospitals announce their new wing or their state of the art new facilities, but they fail to disclose how much their services will cost! No menu!

It is total and complete bullshit that hospitals keep adding to our cost by beautifying their facilities, as people still die of cancer and they still serve their processed foods to the sick and dying! I would rather go to a poll barn with a cure than a fancy hospital with no solutions for me.

We don't like to hear the truth sometimes, but that fact is we are a society looking for easy cures and we will go to many lengths to justify and continue our food addiction. Why? Because like any drug, it feels good and comforts us, but food addiction is worst of all- due to the fact that it doesn't have immediate side effects. Excessive bad foods slowly rot away at us and in the end, we end up decrepit and sick long before our time. This is not normal! In John Robbins wonderful book, Healthy at 100, he explores this subject in detail. Once you read Johns book you will change your mind set about what is normal aging.

Summary from day 26:

30 ounces of vegetable juice (mixed many things): 400

Broccoli and pasta: 400

Lots of raw vegetables: 300

1 Peach: 200

Total calories: 1300

Exercise: Alec and I had a great day of biking and swimming

Thoughts from the day: Great day with my son Alec. We swam in a wonderful creek and biked all over the place. When we got back to his house, we ate a bunch of raw vegetables and a couple of peaches.

DAY: 27

WEIGHT: DID NOT WEIGH IN
DATE: AUGUST 23, 2016

"It is my view that the vegetarian manner of living, by its purely physical effect on the human temperament, would most beneficially influence the lot of mankind." Albert Einstein

It is my 4th day in Golden Colorado, and I am loving life. I am with my son, his girlfriend Alli and his good friend Tyler. They all decided to transfer schools to Denver. From New York (Alec and Alli) and Indiana (Tyler). They wanted to relocate to a better climate and live an active, healthy lifestyle. I am proud of them for making it happen.

Today as I was biking, walking and enjoying the Denver climate, I thought: "Do we want to be a burden on our children as we grow older? If reducing caloric intake can greatly increase your chances of longevity and a quality life than wouldn't it make sense to adopt this behavior? Isn't it our responsibility to conquer our food addiction for the survival of the planet? I guess the question is, do you believe it?

Although- this book is a journal, not a scientific research book. However, I can assure you it is true that your path to a longer, better quality life, is by minimizing food intake and eating highly nutritional foods. Nobody wants to be a burden on our children or society as we grow older?

You cannot help but notice the trillion dollar supplement and weight loss industry advertised all over the place. No doubt, unhealthy people is a good money maker.

Summary from day 27:

16 ounces of green vegetable juice from a juice bar: 300

Large salad: 400

Lots of raw vegetables: 300

Total calories: 1000

Exercise: About 10 miles of walking and a bike ride.

Thoughts from today: Sadly I got a call that my good friend Eric passed away at his home amongst family and friends at about 7 pm today. I am greatly saddened but relieved that he is in no more pain. I regret not being there by his side. I move on with my quest. Eric will never be forgotten.

DAY: 28

WEIGHT: DID NOT WEIGH IN
DATE: AUGUST 24, 2016

"The only way you get that fat off is to eat less and exercise more." Jack LaLanne

Jack LaLanne was a lifelong experiment. This man ate low on the food chain and was an exercise guru but as he got older, he greatly reduced his caloric intake and lived a quality life well in to his late 90s. What a positive influence he was on millions and a benchmark to successful living.

Eating less gives our bodies the ability to heal and allows the body to maximize the nutrients you provide to it. Our digestive systems, like a car engine, need to be treated gently, the oil needs changing and sometimes it just needs to sit still.

Summary from day 28:

Hell day of travel and went off track.

Total calories: Estimated 1400

Exercise: None

Thoughts from today: I had a hellish day of traveling back from Denver by airplane and honestly do not remember much of what I ate but It was all plant based, if you can call airport food that. These days will happen from time to time. One just needs to plan better.

DAY: 29

WEIGHT: 192
DATE: AUGUST 25, 2016

"Your eyes are the eyes of the Universe!" Deepak Chopra

Shockingly I weighed myself and I am two pounds lighter than when I left on my trip to Colorado. I am saddened to be away from that playground but happy to be back to my normal routine. However, I am incredibly sad that I was not able to be by my friend Eric's death bed when he passed on.

Today I aim to get right back on track with juicing and salad only until I reach my goal of 160 to 170 pounds. I did not write much when I was on my trip as I just did not have the thoughts with being so busy.

I have always thought that eating something with eyes is a weird thing. Not to say I have not been hypocritical in doing so but since the age of 12, 80% of my diet has been eyeless. If Deepak is correct with his observations, and I happen to agree, then wouldn't all eyes be connected as one? Thus, if we eat animals- in a sense we are eating ourselves. Therefore, this is cannibalism?

I believe food has different levels of consciousness and what you eat becomes you. As an example: if you eat too much cow and her milk, you will become fat, docile and slow but with animals it goes much further. You are also eating an animal's soul and many times this soul has been corrupted by the insanely cruel world of being raised in a factory for slaughter. Thus, when you consume that, it becomes your body to an extent or at least until your body rejuvenates itself.

One could argue that if our bodies become what we eat, then if one eats a lot of brown rice, wouldn't one become like brown rice? I guess the answer is yes but what is brown rice? Brown rice has no eyes, and its one purpose is to nourish you. It comes from the earth that comes from the universe and the universe is you, isn't it? It seems insane to think, despite what bible thumpers may argue, that animals were put on this planet for us to eat, hunt, torture and wear? I believe animals are us, manifested in a different physical form. No more, no less.

If I am accused of being biased towards vegetarianism, then so be it. This is something that has always felt natural to me and takes little effort. I was raised in a home were eating animals was normal, so I had no real environmental factors that influenced me. One day, I just was.

Like any addiction, we feel comfort from the foods we consume. This addiction, however, unlike valium, as an example, slowly kills us and many times is masked in attractive packaging and advertisers make it look appealing.

Food can be sneaky. It can lurk in the shadows as we go about our daily activities. All the while, working its way through your bloodstream and slowly killing you. You feel tired and do not know why. As you age, you chalk it up and say, "Aging is a bitch." On the other hand, many have chosen a healthier lifestyle and enjoy riding a bike, active sex lives, etc.in to their 90s. It is not unusual on ski slopes, as an example, to see people in their 90s attacking the slopes as many get committed to nursing homes at too young an age and choke down a typical meal of yogurt, apple sauce and hormone infested chicken breast.

Summary from day 29:

16 ounces of beat, lime, apple, cucumber and ginger root: 300

16 ounce banana, strawberry and raspberry smoothie. 300

Large salad with seeds: 400

Avocado and lettuce: 300

Total calories: 1300

Exercise: 75 push-ups and sit-sups

Thoughts from today: Eric was in my thoughts all day today. He was only 44 and I was thinking how lucky I am to have known him.

DAY: 30

WEIGHT: 192
DATE: AUGUST 26, 2016

"Freedom is a place, an area. It's a higher place. There are some other people that are here, and things that are here which are unseen. But you first have to set yourself free and believe in what you cannot see, believe that there is something more out there. In freedom can be found many devotions: a devotion to love, a desire to believe, a willingness to be happy, and a perseverance to have peace. All these unseen things breathe and grow in the unseen soul. A free person is not an uncommitted person, but in a free person you will find a deep devotion, and a desire to be devoted to even more." Joy Bell

I do believe that a fast can offer one a sense of enlightenment and freedom from the slavery of food. By writing down my thoughts each day I am developing a higher appreciation for food and water. Food and water are life giving and I think we have lost our respect for it all together, but it is not our faults. It is the faults of manufactures and advertisers that push snake oil on us. Deceptive studies, charts and advertising designed to increase the bottom line as the people of America suffer with and all time high obesity rate and unspeakable health issues. It is time we change, isn't it?

Don't you think most of us settle in as we age and have preconceived expectations? We expect to be tired. We are expected to lose our sex drive. We expect to get sick. That is what they want! That mindset is a big money maker! It is almost as if "they" want us sick for profit. There is not much profit in eating significantly less and healthier bodies, is there? Eating less offers you premium health and major costs savings. So why wouldn't we all do it? First, we do not believe it! Second, we have not confronted the fact that we have an addiction.

To reiterate, there is no need to live at a gym when you are fully conscious of what you eat and the amount you eat. You will no longer feel guilty when you miss a workout, nor waste money on expensive health club memberships. You will no longer have the need to eat useless sweets and animal foods.

Tonight, will be a difficult task as Eric will be laid to rest. No doubt, once again, there will be beer and cheer to celebrate his life. There will be plenty of comfort food offerings, masked as warm and fuzzy but I know different. I know that the mac and cheese, sweets, pulled pork, fried chicken, cold cuts, cream based dips - all contributed to Eric's early exit from this life. Eric was full of joy and loved life. He was only 44.

Below is Eric's obituary but trust me, it hardly gives his life justice. We had intimate talks together and Eric was trying to change his diet and exercise program, but I am afraid it came too late.

Eric was diagnosed on January 15, 2016 and died only 7 months later. I spoke with him about a massive juice cleansing, but his doctor's advice superseded mine and who am I, with no fancy titles, only well-read and common sense, to compete with ole Doc? Eric did, and I helped, purchase a genuinely nice road bicycle but the chemo and pills did not allow him to ride much. He continued with the meat consumption and people continued to bring him "comfort foods" that we know, contribute to all cancers. But people have great intentions! Again, it all goes back to mind control from birth.

Eric was strong. He battled this shit to the end, and I have never seen anything like it. If there is anyone, I would want to be in a fox hole with, it was Eric, and therefore I will continue my quest at a feverish pace.

In short, it pisses me the fuck off that we have all this knowledge, but we are too fucking lazy to do anything about it. Even facing death, Eric was fed these foods that accelerated his death. Even when hospitalized, the comfort foods kept coming. Doctors and nurses should be ashamed that this is the norm. Hate me, if you will but my goal is not to placate to anyone but to get them to think. If you want to be comforted, go see a priest or typical doctor in America who will tell you what you want to hear.

Eric Robert Kehrt, 44, of Plainfield, passed away August 23, 2016. He was born December 25, 1971 in Indianapolis, IN. He was a 1990 graduate of Emeriti Manual High School. He was currently a commercial equipment installer for C&T Designs for the past 21 years. He was active in coaching Little League football, basketball and baseball in Plainfield. For recreation he loved fishing and disc golf. Eric is survived by his wife, Lisa M. (Lutz) Kart. They were married on September 17, 1994. He is also survived by two sons, Tyler R. and Ryan E. Kart; his mother, Sheila Candler; father and step-mother, Phillip and Liz Kart; grandfather, Charles Swan; grandmother, Evelyn Beavers; brother, Don Kart; and a sister Jenny (Josh) Lee. Visitation will be from 4:00 to 8:00 pm on Friday, August 26, 2017 in the Hampton-Gentry Funeral Home, Plainfield. Memorial services will be at 1:00 pm on Saturday, August 27 in the funeral home, with calling one hour prior to services.

Summary from day 30:

16 ounce beet, lime, ginger and cucumber juice: 300

16 ounce banana, strawberry smoothie: 300

1 huge salad with seeds and some fresh fruits and vegetables: 600

Total calories: 1200

Exercise: 30 minutes of walking and 50 push-ups and sit-ups

Thoughts from my bike ride: Sometimes I juice what's available and just try and be economical about it.

DAY: 31
WEIGHT: 191
DATE: AUGUST 27, 2016

"Death ends a life, not a relationship." Mitch Albom

Last night was a difficult time. My friend Eric now passed on from this life. Eric was cremated. At the service, there were a nice assortment of pictures and videos that represented his life. Luckily for me, I was part of many of those more recent memories of his life.

At the funeral home, kind people and the Boosters Club brought in an assortment of veggie trays, bean salads and other somewhat healthier selections for people to munch on. However, a smorgasbord of cold cuts, cheeses, white breads and soda became the star attraction. Once again, the irony is that meat and dairy products contribute greatly to cancer.

When you think outside the box, as with a massive dietary change, you will no doubt face great opposition. You will be accused of having an eating disorder or perhaps being a freak. But I assure you this is no different than any radical idea or change that has taken place in the history of the world. People simply do not know any better. As I have repeatedly said, they have been brainwashed since birth to eat a certain way, so it is not easy to break bad habits.

It is getting easier to say no to food that is made by family members as I explain to them that I am giving my body a break. You must learn to say no in a polite manner, or you will not fully retrain your mind. Eat when you want, what you want and when you want. Perhaps this thinking contradicts the perceived value of "family dinner time" but I think you as an individual have a basic human right to eat what makes you feel good, regardless of hurt feelings.

We talk about food disorders but continually eat excessive calories. That is not addiction? How can this be possible? If we center just about everything we do around food, how is this not a disorder? I feel that food addiction is the number one addiction in our country and the number one destroyer of health, self-esteem, relationships and the planet. This is a fact we refuse to acknowledge. In fact, there will be a barrage of criticism against this book to justify food addiction once again.

Summary from day 31:

16 ounce carrot, apple, lime, lettuce and tomato juice: 300

16 ounce banana and strawberry smoothie: 300

Huge salad with seeds and piece of bread: 600

Totals calories: 1000

Exercise: 13 mile bike ride.

Thoughts from my bike ride: Keep pushing on!

DAY: 32

WEIGHT: 189
DATE: AUGUST 28, 2016

"You have just dined, and however scrupulously the slaughterhouse is concealed in the graceful distance of miles, there is complicity." Ralph Waldo Emerson

Food comes in colorful packaging that is sold at a colorful place, so we are far removed from its origin. If we knew of its origin we would think twice before eating it.

Today I am another 2 pounds down and cruising. This is no doubt a result of eating less calories and nutritious foods.

I want to be clear that food is a fantastic aspect of life, but food should be simple, natural and eaten with respect. Complicated recipes that contain high fat animal products and processed ingredients should be kept to a minimum.

Fasting is not for those that have an eating disorder, and I am hardly qualified to elaborate on this subject, but most people simply eat too many calories.

Summary from day 32:

32 ounce carrot, cucumber, lime, green pepper juice: 500

Large salad: 350

Total calories: 850

Exercise: 13 mile bike ride.

Thoughts from my bike ride: Yesterday we said goodbye to Eric and had a nice get together at an Italian restaurant. Once again, the meat and cheese were ordered in abundance. I could not help but notice.

DAY: 33

WEIGHT: 188
DATE: AUGUST 29, 2016

"John Candy knew he was going to die. He told me on his 40th birthday. He said, well, Maureen, I'm on borrowed time." Maureen O'Hara

Most who grew up with John Candy, a big man, can chuckle at the above quote. He obviously, as the above quote suggest, knew that the way he lived would not afford him longevity in life. As many Americans do, he probably was suffering from food addiction.

In the moment, comfort food feels good to us but rapidly what we eat becomes a sense of guilt and a multitude of other ailments can follow. So how does one stop, begin to change her ways? Personally, I simply think you take one step, you fast for 1 day and start a journal of what you eat. You eliminate anything that is processed from your diet. The first step is the hardest step, but it will get easier each day.

Eric lived life with passion. He loved beer, going out to dinner and he loved his 2 boys and wife more than anyone will ever know. He loved talking sports. He did not talk bad about anyone and he was a loyal friend.

For many of us we cannot see that meat and dairy products are death, masked pretty by the ones who profit. To grow, you must sit and ponder deeper from what you see in front of you.

Some may insist that food is food, and it is all about genes and luck. That the idea of food addiction is absurd. But to me, that is a measure of how numb we have become. We have grown a "second skin". But when we get sick or lay on our death beds, it is a major kick in the ass.

Summary from day 33:

16 ounce carrot, lime and apple juice: 300

16 ounce banana and strawberry smoothie: 300

Large salad and a baked potato: 500

Total calories: 1100

Exercise: 14 mile bike ride. 50 push-ups.

Thoughts from my bike ride: This is day 33. My body is transforming but I still have over 25 pounds to lose until my goal of 160. I am not sure I will make that goal.

DAY: 34

WEIGHT: 188
DATE: AUGUST 30, 2016

"The greatest enemy of hunger for God is not poison but apple pie.

It is not the banquet of the wicked that dulls our appetite for heaven, but endless nibbling at the table of the world. It is not the X-rated video, but the prime-time dribble of triviality we drink in every night." John Piper, a Hunger for God

To fast is not easy. As soon as we feel that first hunger of the day it is so easy to eat to kill the pain by eating. Or is it pain? I think it is just are programming and like any addiction, we reach for a substance to get rid of the pain. So how do we fast? I do not know the answer other than will power.

Just sitting still and observing the world around us is enough sometimes for change to occur. This technique has been successful for me on many occasions. I think thoughts and they become things. I have too many examples to list. All existence is connected, and your thoughts reach out as energy to anything connected to you.

I wanted to be clear that when I first started this, I had no intention of a "juice fast" until I saw the movie Fat Sick, and Almost Dead but it seemed like a good idea. My goal for life, is to eat a calorie restricted diet consisting of mostly plant based whole foods.

Summary from day 34:

3 juiced oranges and a tomato: 250

Tomato soup: 150

Peanut butter sandwich: 350

Wheat pasta: 250

Total calories: 1000

Exercise: 10 mile bike ride.

Thoughts from my bike ride: Today I am transforming a little. I will juice continually as I am convinced of the benefits but add 1 solid meal a day and continue to count calories.

DAY: 35

WEIGHT: 188
DATE: AUGUST 31, 2016

"Our love of being right is best understood as our fear of being wrong" Kathryn Schulz

The eating animal's debate is no debate at all. If, in fact, we were designed to eat meat wouldn't we simply, as other animals, just climb on a cow and start eating? Sure, we cab virtually eat anything so why not choose optimal health choices such as whole-plant based foods? This question has virtually blown me away since as early as I can remember. I think the answer is simple. We simply do not think and are selfish in our ways. We want what we want and furthermore, if we appear healthy, what we do not see does not bother us and we stop when it's too late.

There are people we all know, maybe even you, that still believe that what we eat has extraordinarily little to do with health, longevity, disease and its impact on the environment. That it is all a crap shoot, all luck, genes. They think, "When the "maker" calls your name that's it- nothing you can do." But there are those of us, me included, that find this thinking to be barbaric, ignorant and frankly stupid.

Bottom line, if you want to age well then eat a plant based diet with lots of variety and you will have a much greater chance to see your grandchildren grow and not be a burden on them. If not, you are trading in common sense for your senseless need to eat fried chicken wings and steak.

We all think we are invincible when we feel good but how quickly that shifts when we are on our death beds. How quickly do we regret those stupid choices we made?

Summary from day 35:

Oatmeal and bananas: 300

Brown rice and vegetables: 400

16 ounce carrot and apple juice: 300

Total calories: 1000

Exercise: 20 mile bike ride. 50 push-ups. 50 sit-ups.

Thoughts from my bike ride: How many woman and men lie in bed dullened by life, night after night as their bodies rot slowly from the heavy meat and cheeses, they have consumed. The good news is you can quickly turn this around. Our bodies heal at a rapid pace when given the right fuel.

DAY: 36

WEIGHT: 187
DATE: SEPTEMBER 1, 2016

"Fall seven times, stand up eight." Japanese Proverb

I have always been health conscious but up until now I have never tried anything as strict as this. I think the key is keeping a journal. What you eat becomes vividly clear when you write it down each day and it keeps you accountable. Seeing it in writing seems to have an impact and I believe that is helping my success. Also, I am re-programing my mind of 53 years of food impressions from my parents, doctors, teachers, food pyramids and advertisers.

I do not think I have ever had a fast metabolism, so I must be patient. At 53 I likely have a metabolic rate slower than a person in their 30s but faster than a person in their 70s. I aim for this to be my new way of eating. Hopefully, a few people who read this book will benefit as I have.

Yes, I am suggesting you take extreme measures in changing your diet, but I am confident that it will be well worth it. You will watch your children grow and their children grow. You will age gracefully and be well capable in your later years. You will not be a burden on our failing health care system, and you will have a positive impact on the environment. So, if you were guaranteed this, would you do it? Well, the encouraging news is millions before us have taken this leap and there are thousands of studies to show this to be true. For me, being a decent vegetarian most of my life has afforded me solid health with not many ailments or hospital visits. But stepping it up to another level, has given me a new vitality and outlook on life.

*For the record: I have cheated extraordinarily little on this diet, but I have been weakened by temptation on a few occasions with a handful of chips here, a bite of rice there and a taste of this or that not to offend someone. But over the years, to my regret, I certainly have offended many with my snide gestures or tone of voice over the years when it came to offerings or food choices. The insignificant amounts of processed foods ingested over the last 36 days were too infrequent and minuscule to record and probably did not add up to more than 500 calories total. However, on the other hand, I have been conservative with my bike riding estimates and added a few calories to my daily intakes. You will never find a perfect formula, but it is important to stay within range of estimates when trying to reach a goal. But please do not beat yourself up if you dabble in a few foods here and there.

Summary from day 36:

16 ounce carrot and apple juice: 300

Vegetable/bean burger on an oat bun with a side salad: 500

Total calories: 800

Exercise: 11 mile bike ride.

Thoughts from my bike ride: I have transformed to mostly carrot and apple juice as it is inexpensive, juices easily and taste good. I do not know what optimal juice is, nobody really does but it makes good sense to have variety in your diet of whole foods.

For me, common sense is that you keep it simple, but you will never find the "perfect" diet. But I can tell you that my personal experiment here is working great so I can safely assume, since we are all similar biologically, that it will work for you as it has for thousands before us.

DAY: 37

WEIGHT: 186
DATE: SEPTEMBER 2, 2016

"Cultivate solitude and quiet and a few sincere friends, rather than mob merriment, noise and thousands of nodding acquaintances." William Powell

Being a vegetarian most of my life has brought much criticism and questions. I have learned to keep quieter and sometimes just placate to people to avoid conversation all together. I have found that sometimes it is not worth my time to waste. But by my example, I have slowly transformed many who have known me into non-flesh eating people. Through example much can be accomplished.

During my time living in New Mexico in the 1990s, I hosted a public broadcast show called Ask the Vegetarian. The premise of the show was simple. I would invite guest on the show and the public could call in live to discuss the pros and cons of being a vegetarian. The show ran for about a year, once a week and was successful.

Back in those days I was much more vocal about my passions. But then again, it was Albuquerque NM, where people were much more liberal than Indiana. Living in Indiana, a meat eating mecca, has kept my mouth quieter.

When I was a kid growing up in Massachusetts, I remember people in my quiet town of Needham being more health conscious than today's modern world. It appears society has gone backwards. Too much fast food, too much processed food, too much junk food, too much!

Today I feel good and am holding steady at under 190 pounds. Sadly, it has been about 3 years since I have been under that mark but prior to that, most of my adult life, I usually fluctuated between about 175 and 190 pounds. I have always eaten too much. So, this newfound diet of mine is not just about what I eat but the amounts.

I have started wearing some of my son's clothes. I have been no smaller than an XL to XXL in most shirts and my waste has been between 36 and 40 for the last three years. My son wears a large shirt and a 33 to 34 inch pant size. I am 5'10" compared to his 6'2" slim frame. I guess you could call me stalky now but that is hardly my "body style". I feel like a have a natural athletic body style (wide shoulders, big hands and feet) and I feel as though, even at 53, I am well on my way back to it. It is a great feeling to wear clothes that fit better-a real confidence builder. To me, what the scale says is not as fulfilling as how my clothes fit. Love it!

Summary from day 37:

16 ounce carrot and apple juice: 300

Veggie burger plain: 150

Glass of orange juice: 150

Some hummus and stone ground chips: 300

Baked potato: 200

Total calories: 1100

Exercise: 75 push-ups. 12 mile bike ride.

Thoughts from my bike ride: Adding some solid foods has been an easy transition but the challenge is, like last night, too many social gatherings offer too much crap. Thus- it is important to bring your own healthier choices.

DAY: 38
WEIGHT: 187
DATE: SEPTEMBER 3, 2016

"I was not created to be occupied by eating delicious foods like tied up cattle." Ali ibn Abi Talib

When I attempted this last year, I failed quickly. I started during the holidays in the dead of winter and I thought because I am a vegetarian that it would be easy, but I was wrong.

Saying no to meat and dairy products is a step in the right direction but saying yes to only whole-plant based foods is the way. What is a whole food then? Anything that has been unchanged from its original form is a whole food.

I weighed in at 187 this morning and now I am 25 pounds down in just 38 days without much sacrifice at all.

When I feel hungry, it is a good feeling and my energy levels have never been better. The only thing I have done is make a conscious effort to eat significantly less calories of nutrient rich whole foods.

By writing down my progress and keeping myself accountable, I have easily shed weight. You could call this a scientific approach or a spiritual approach. Whatever you call it, losing weight is clearly and equation of burning more calories than you take in.

Summary from day 38:

16 ounce banana and strawberry smoothie: 300

Black beans, onions, fresh jalapeno and stone ground chips: 400

Veggie burger: 300

16 ounces of carrot and apple juice: 300

Total calories: 1300

Exercise: 20 miles on bike. 50 push-ups.

Thoughts from my bike ride: I was thinking on my bike ride that the entire "snack concept" is a little odd. What is a snack really? It seems we have become so programed that as soon as we feel the least bit of hunger we reach for a snack. Those initial hunger pains are just animal instincts telling you to eat more for more fat storage. We all know that if you just wait a bit or drink a glass of water, we can get over those hunger pains until the next sensible meal.

Most of us have been accustomed to including "snacks" in our plans when we go on a trip. It appears we would benefit more if we learned to get through those initial hunger pains. Simply learn to grab an apple or handful of almonds. The "snack" food industry is profiting off our weaknesses, making billions as type 2 diabetes leaches on to more and more people-our children!

Charles Caprarella

Let us be honest, most "snacks" are not even food at all but a "food product". Just because a food product lists nutrients does not mean it is good for you. Nutrient selling-marketing is nothing more than political lobbying and has profit in mind, not anyone's health. If you need to snack, choose foods that have no labels and make no health claims.

DAY: 39
WEIGHT: 185
DATE: SEPTEMBER 4, 2016

"We never know which lives we influence, or when, or why."
Stephen King

Books, movies, documentaries and people have influenced me. Those influences are who we become so I think it's important to seek knowledge, question authority and try new things.

I am down to 185 pounds today so with 21 more days to go I am suspecting I will fall short by 15 pounds and end up at 175 or so. I am good with that. But my goal is still to eventually get to 160 pounds and stay there.

Obviously results will vary with each individual. I did not start off on this quest obese or grossly out of shape and I was already eating better than most so the shock on my body was minimal, but my results have been tremendous. My skin has never been healthier, my energy is way up, my sex drive is good, and my overall mood has increased tremendously.

In my life, the people I have met and books I have read have shaped who I am today. Thank goodness I did not follow the path of what society, teachers, doctors, food pyramids taught me when it came to food choices. When I first told my parents, I was becoming a vegetarian at 12 they laughed at me and said, you cannot do that because you will become skinny, frail and break bones. Interestingly I became a 3 sport athlete and excelled at football, baseball and basketball and alas, never broke a bone. In fact, gaining weight and muscle for me was always easy on my non-animal based diet. Albeit, I was eating a lot of pizza and French fries, along with many healthier choices, apparently, we function fine without animal foods.

I am not alone. Billions of people for thousands of years have excelled on a mostly plant based diet so why all the fuss about eat your meat and drink your milk for strong bones? Well, this is common sense. It is for money and money only! In the must read book, Diet for a New America, John Robbins goes into detail about this truth. All Mr. Robbins books are a must read.

Summary from day 39:

16 ounce carrot and apple juice: 300

Mixed fruits: 300

Black beans and corn chips: (large portion): 600

16 ounce banana and strawberry smoothie: 300

Total calories: 1500

Exercise: 50 push ups

Thoughts from today: I went to a get together today amongst friends in observances of Labor Day. Of course, meat was grilling, and the mayo based salads and high caloric sweets were offered in abundance but fortunately there was a lot of fruit available.

This has just become the "norm" in America so one has to be prepared for these times. I drank 2 lite beers and enjoyed the day with good friends. When I got home, I made some black beans and scooped them with organic stone ground chips. Tomorrow is another day!

I have gotten so accustomed to watching others gorge on hamburgers hot dogs and cream based dishes that I am almost numb to it. Many times, I feel like I am from another planet.

DAY: 40

WEIGHT: 186
DATE: SEPTEMBER 5, 2016

"Remember that guy that gave up? Neither does no one else."
Unknown

I have never really thought about giving up on this journey but for the record, I have failed many times in life. But I have had many successes as well. I only have 20 more days to go and can do this!

This is the first day in 40 days that I weigh more (1 pound) than I did the day before.

I will say again that the key to this program's success is accountability. By writing down my thoughts each day I have retrained my subconscious mind.

The point here is not to have to force weight loss by working out obsessively or having to feel like you are sacrificing the foods you love. Cutting back on calories allows your body to heal and re-shape itself. Feeling slimmer and healthier has endless benefits both seen and unseen. When you eat less, you not only help yourself, but you also help the environment and help curb world hunger.

Charles Caprarella

Summary from day 40:

Half of a banana: 100

Thai Green Salad: 300

Bowl of Brown rice: 300

16 ounce carrot and apple juice: 300

Total calories: 1000

Exercise: 14 mile bike ride. 50 push-ups. 50 sit-ups.

Thoughts from my bike ride: I was thinking how I have been to one too many funerals as of late for 2 people that died way before their time. Brian, a 49 year old husband and father of two died suddenly of a massive heart attack at his home. Apparently, the autopsy revealed heavily blocked arties. Brian was a fun loving guy and at his funeral the priest and friends-relatives delivered great speeches about how much Brian loved life and how he loved his beer and good times. However, no mention of what caused the sudden heart attack. Eric, my good buddy, died 7 months after a cancer diagnoses at the age of 44. At his funeral there was no mention of what could have been the culprit of early death.

I am not suggesting that if Eric and Brian had been vegan, maintained healthier weight and drank more moderately that they would still be around to see their kids and grandchildren grow up, but overwhelming statistics would have been in their favor.

What is startling to me is that people go to church on Sunday and hear extraordinarily little about health. Instead, they hear the priest confidently preach, "your time is up when your maker calls for you" and there is little explanation for suffering other than it is a mystery or god is testing you. Hmm-curious if you ask me.

DAY: 41

WEIGHT: 185
DATE: SEPTEMBER 6, 2016

"I know for sure what we dwell on is who we become." Oprah Winfrey

Society does not want you wise. It is not in society's best interest for you to be wise. It is in society's best interest for you to be obedient and not question authority. It is in the grave digger's best interest for you to not ask questions.

I will be wrapping this book up at day 60, regardless of my weight. I have gone long enough to know that eating this way will shed pounds and heal you. No need to drag it on and bore the reader. Fact is, it works. If you want to live a long and healthy life this is it, right in front of you. You just need to start today.

First step go buy a vegetable juicer and some fresh vegetables and juice only for at least two weeks, and then start calorie counting and write down your intake each day. You will achieve similar results.

Many will tell you that counting calories does not work and that may be true to an extent. However, what is failed to mention is that population growth is out of control and eating less is not just about you, it's about everyone's survival.

Summary from day 41:

16 ounces of carrot, apple, celery and ginger juice: 300

16 ounce banana and strawberry smoothie: 300

Large salad: 350

Total calories: 950

Exercise: 10 mile bike ride. 50 sit-ups. 50 push-ups.

Thoughts from my bike ride: It was very hot today, 90 degrees with 75% humidly. Sweating felt good and cooled me down but I am not a fan of humidity.

DAY: 42

WEIGHT: 184
DATE: SEPTEMBER 7, 2016

"Obstacles don't have to stop you. If you run into a wall, don't turn around and give up. Figure out how to climb it, go through it, or work around it." Michael Jordan

I have faced many obstacles on this journey. Overcoming the negativity of others, social gatherings, easy access to fast food, to name a few.

For years I thought certain processed and boxed food were on the healthy side but now my thinking has changed. Anything, processed, including soy and vegan foods should be consumed minimally.

Fair warning, you will truly be the minority if you decide to adopt this lifestyle so strap yourself in and get ready for a ride.

It's a somewhat lonely road too, unless you belong to a support group or have someone that will do it with you. I wish I did sometimes, but I do well on my own.

But obstacles make us stronger as we develop resiliency and a no quit attitude. How many of us started out on a diet but quickly we go off it because of the influences around us? Maybe someone brings home a bag of chips or orders pizza or invites us out for dinner, knowing we are trying hard to change our ways? This is just the way it is, and we must stand our ground.

For me, I just keep reminding myself that I am done living a life of compromise and damn it, this is my body I must live with. It is the only one I will ever have! But it would be nice if this were normal. In contrast its normal, to eat fast food, cheeseburgers and candy! Sadly, this is the reality right now in our society.

I am at 184 pounds today. I wish I could say, I never felt better but I still have a long way to go. Seeing results is a great motivator. It appears the fresh vegetable juice, even with some solid foods, is continually, slowly, eliminating waste from my body and even sort of melting away the excess's fat. I am fascinated by how it is working.

Let us face it, there are many diets that help you lose weight but this one feels so natural and clean. Of course, I will face criticism but I have lived it so there is not much someone could say to discourage me. I am sure critics will say that it is unrealistic, and it will not last. Of course, like any diet, I know I will gain some weight back but hopefully I can continue to stay out of the hospitals and off pills. As I have stated before, it is not just about weight.

Summary from day 42:

16 ounce carrot, beat, apple and ginger juice: 300

10 ounce cucumber, lime and tomato apple juice: 200

Black beans and onion: 400

Mixed salad: 300

Total calories: 1200

Exercise: 13 mile bike ride. 50 push-ups. 50 sit-ups.

Thoughts from my bike ride: I am content with my results and feel good, but I am not satisfied yet. I weighed in at 184 pounds today, so that is 26 pounds lost in 42 days. But there is a part of me that said, "How the hell did it come to this." I mean to say, how does a vegetarian, health conscious person get 50 pounds overweight? The only excuse I have is I just slowly took on eating too much processed and high fat foods. But one must not dwell on the past, one must live in the moments!

DAY: 43
WEIGHT: 184
DATE: SEPTEMBER 8, 2016

"Any fool can make a rule and any fool will mind it." Henry
David Thoreau

Who made the rules on what to eat and how much to eat?
It is a complicated question, but I think we can give much
of the blame to the almighty meat and dairy industries. We
all remember that food pyramid poster hanging in schools
and doctors' offices. This heavily funded and manipulating
scheme has but one goal, to sell more shit to us for profit. So
how evil and manipulating is all this propaganda on what
to eat? It is up there with the worst of all evils ever to exist.

Nowadays we know damn well we do not need milk for
strong bones and meat for protein and that a whole food-
plant based diet is a superior choice so why is milk and
meat still in our schools? The answer is simply money, the
almighty buck!

We must be skeptical of recipes that require baking,
sautéing, frying, heavy creams, butter, milk, cheese and

meat because most of these fancy dishes do your body no good, are expensive and time consuming to make. Dishes like that have a negative impact on your body and the environment, not to mention they contribute greatly to the mistreatment of animals.

I recently read a good book, In Defense of Food by Michael Pollan, he suggested we eat nothing with more than 5 ingredients in it or something that has ingredients that we cannot pronounce. That is a good guide but that also suggest that we should choose our processed foods more wisely. I agree, but the goal here is to greatly reduce or eliminate processed foods altogether.

My book suggests radical changes in your dietary lifestyle but think about how this book just 50 years ago would not even have been that radical. This is because at no other time in the history of the world has our food supply been so processed. The grocery stores are evident of this fact and one might only need to spend an hour in a grocery store and observe what people are buying to realize this fact. We have an epidemic and something must be done now, or the health of the people will continue to plummet.

This makes you rethink culinary schools and so called master chefs. Is it all bullshit? The argument would be that food is joyful and should be enjoyed, that fancy prepared foods play a big role in the joy in our lives. Yet the hard cold truth is that many artistic dishes are a pile of shit that destroys our bodies, contributes greatly to all major diseases and helps put us in an early grave. But many will still argue that ole grandad lived to over 100 or so and he ate what he wanted. If insurance companies were to take on this sort of logic, opposed to data, they would be out of business in no time.

We cannot ignore the evil marketing plotted by the advertising agencies to hustle their shit on people. This is way more elaborate of a scheme than the drug dealer because it is designed to brainwash our youth. It is designed to make our youth zombies to the man, slaves to the system.

At the end of the day, food is food, and any food will provide you with energy. Very simply, food gets broken down within your body and becomes who you are. And we are so fortunate to even have a choice what to eat. So, with all we know, in this day and age of knowledge, why not make good food choices that will help us live longer and healthier lives?

Summary from day 43:

16 ounce banana and strawberry smoothie: 300

Huge bowl of veggie stew: 400

Total calories: 700

Exercise: 11 mile bike ride. 50 push-ups. 50 sit-ups.

Thoughts from my bike ride: I was observing all the runners, walkers and bikers and thought how all these people are trying to feel better, lose weight or simply want to enjoy nature. It's always encouraging for me to see people enjoying the simple things in life. I also thought how many, despite exercise, still struggle with weight and health because of their food choices. Exercise is truly not enough, especially as we age, in this world of toxic food choices. Choose your foods wisely!

DAY: 44

WEIGHT: 183
DATE: SEPTEMBER 9, 2016

"The only thing standing between you and your goal is the bullshit story you keep telling yourself as to why you can't achieve it." Jordan Belfort

Quoting a former thief like Belfort has its contradictions with a book like this but what can I say, I liked the movie Wolf of Wall-Street. Apparently, Belfort has since paid for his crimes and changed his ways. However, the quote is true at many levels when it comes to drastically changing one's diet. I here excuses all the time. "I could never give up meat", they say. "My blood sugar drops too low when I don't eat enough." I have heard them all when the topic of eating low on the food chain comes up and/or drastically reducing the number of calories we eat.

I weighed in at 183 today. Many people have commented on me looking thinner, but I haven't discussed this book with many people and I never really looked fat, per say, so the change is coming gradually.

The problem with most diets and exercise plans is that they are temporary. One will join a gym and go a few times a week and lose interest. One will join weight watchers, lose 30 pounds and gain it back.

Diet and exercise cannot be a hobby. To have long term results you must make it your life, not a side note. But sadly, many put their job or other activities as a priority over their health. The solution is to ingrain a healthy lifestyle into your life and make it your number one priority.

Once you start living healthier, others will start to respect your space and time. But you must be prepared not to be a people pleaser and get ready for resistance. Others will attempt to bring you down and say, "a little pizza is ok."

Saying no, as best you can, is the answer. Once you start to say no, you will find over time, that it is who you become. Stand your ground and be stubborn. This is your only life and your only body. Protect it! Do what you must do but stop letting others around you dictate what you eat and how much you eat.

Summary from day 44:

30 ounce carrot, apple and ginger juice: 450

Pretzels at a neighbor's house: 300

Total calories: 750

Exercise: 9 mile bike ride.

Thoughts from my bike ride: When you really think about it, any food sold for profit must be scrutinized. Just watch TV for a few hours and observe the food commercials. Beautiful music, and pleasant images are carefully scripted to sell their clients products to you.

I recently saw a Philadelphia Strawberry Cream Cheese commercial where wonderful images of fresh strawberries were proudly displayed and the narrator is saying, "no artificial flavors used". Moms run out and buy that pasteurized cow piss thinking that they are doing something good for their children. Advertisers lurk like evil thugs in dark allies and prey on your naive mind!

DAY: 45

WEIGHT: 183
DATE: SEPTEMBER 10, 2016

"If you don't know where you are going, you'll end up someplace else." Yogi Berra

Writing down a goal is not enough in itself. An action plan, with a proven track record is needed and therefore this is working for me. I have a basic knowledge of what the caloric content is in most foods and I have a good idea of what it takes each day to maintain my current weight, gain weight or lose weight. The 1200 calorie figure I came up with was thought out but not a scientific formula. I would suggest you just start out with a figure, write down your results each day and adjust as needed.

A 1500 calorie a day maximum for the rest of my life seems to be a good amount for me. Again, it is the quality of calories that is more important than the quantity. Concentrate on highly nutritional whole foods as much as possible. Maybe give yourself a 20% margin of error. This will give you room for some imperfection.

As an example: Studies show that 160 calories from Almonds are absorbed slower than a Pepsi because a Pepsi contains nothing but refined sugar and has no fiber. The fiber allows absorption to be natural, as our bodies are designed. In contrast, refined sugar gets processed immediately and as fat!

Fed Up, Documentary

But there is no perfect number here. So, for those of you who are very analytical, I do not know what to tell you other than there is no such thing as perfection when it comes to these matters. In short, you need to know where you want to go, make a goal, and just start taking those steps in the right direction. Think, "is this food I am going to eat a deposit or a withdrawal."

In the movie Forrest Gump, Forrest was in a deep depression, so he just started running for no apparent reason but by the end, after running thousands of miles, he just stopped and felt better. I know this is fictional but very profound. He was smart enough to know the cure but not smart enough to question it. Do not argue with your gut instinct is the moral because it is hardly ever wrong.

I find it hard to eat something with eyes. Again, we cannot escape cruelty as all things live. But the plant foods we eat become part of us. I find it a form of cannibalism to eat things with eyes. As an example: Pigs share several surprising comparable traits with humans. For instance, we both have some hairless skin, a thick layer of subcutaneous fat, light-colored eyes, protruding noses and heavy eyelashes. Pig skin tissues and heart valves can be used in medicine because of their compatibility with the human body. But this is just one example of multitudes.

This is most likely why dead animals make one feel so, well, dead. We nap off the turkey flesh at thanksgiving and during that nap the death of the turkey both physically and its spirit ravish its way around our bloodstream. This is very confusing to our organs and soul. On the other hand, Hitler was a vegetarian so I might be called out on that vivid contrast. However, as we examine cultures, plant eaters tend to be less aggressive, enjoy better relationships and health. Would there be less war, arguments, etc., if the world were mostly vegan?

We lovingly tell our children to wash their hands free of dirt, but we think nothing of them licking their cute little fingers coated with animal blood as they eat their ribs! Ridiculous, isn't it?

Charles Caprarella

Summary from day 45:

28 ounces of carrot, apple and celery juice: 400

Small mixed greens salad and a piece of bread: 300

2 heavy beers and potato salad at a German Festival: 600

Total calories: 1300

Exercise: 12 mile bike ride. 100 push-ups. 50 sit-ups.

Thoughts from my bike ride: None of us could ever eat perfectly all the time but I think it is realistic to shoot for at least 80% of our diets to consist of unprocessed foods.

DAY: 46

WEIGHT: 183
DATE: SEPTEMBER 11, 2016

"The carnistic schema, which twists information so that nonsense seems to make perfect sense, also explains why we fail to see the absurdities of the system. Consider, for instance, advertising campaigns in which a pig dances joyfully over the fire pit where he or she is to be barbecued, or chickens wear aprons while beseeching the viewer to eat them. And consider the Veterinarian's Oath of the American Veterinary Medical Association, 'I solemnly swear to use my...skills for the...relief of animal suffering,' in light of the fact that the vast majority of veterinarians eat animals simply because they like the way meat tastes. Or think about how people won't replace their hamburgers with veggie burgers, even if the flavor is identical, because they claim that, if they try hard enough, they can detect a subtle difference in texture. Only when we deconstruct the carnistic schema can we see the absurdity of placing our preference for a flawless re-creation of a textural norm over the lives and deaths of billions of others." Melanie Joy, Why We Love Dogs, Eat Pigs, and Wear Cows: An Introduction to Carnism: The Belief System That Enables Us to Eat Some Animals and Not Others

People love their cats and dogs but think nothing of a baby cow masked as veal cutlet or a spring lamb masked as a delicious delicacy or the baby back rib that had no chance to cuddle with mom. Yet multitudes feverishly defend against abortion and the right to life. Absurd.

It is estimated by the national cancer foundation that cooking food at high temperatures, especially meat, can greatly increase your cancer risk. So, isn't it wise to choose raw foods whenever you can? I am not saying never cook but a wise man would not. Yet, we gather at cookouts by the millions each weekend as charred cow and processed pig sizzles in their own blood, as children play joyfully.

The true gage of health should not be weight or visuals. After all, multitudes of thin people are unhealthy, and many heavier people are vibrant and energetic. Visuals can sway us and are dangerous. Example, a thin person eats whatever they want and are proud of that fact. They confidently say, "I eat what I want so it must be all genetics." However, this is dangerous as it represents a small percentage of the people. I believe if you study people over 40, as life has started to take its toll, you will find that despite weight, the diet they keep will be in direct correlation to doctor visits, ailments, pill popping and overall energy and sex drive.

Summary from day 46:

20 ounce banana, blueberry and strawberry smoothie: 350

16 ounce carrot, beat, ginger, celery and lemon juice: 300

Large mixed salad: 400

Total calories: 950

Exercise: 15 mile bike ride. 100 push-ups. 50 sit-ups.

Thoughts from my bike: Soda is gross, I agree! For me, I am working on eliminating it from my life as I drink about one diet soda a day. This is the hypocrisy I formerly mentioned, as if we search, we are all guilty at times. But I want to reiterate that I do not think I am better than anyone else. In this little book, I am simply spilling my thoughts out on these pages as they come each day and you the reader, can take the good and the bad. Although, I am hopeful you will gain something to think about from reading it.

DAY: 47

WEIGHT: DID NOT WEIGH IN
DATE: SEPTEMBER 12, 2016

"If slaughterhouses had glass walls, everyone would be a vegetarian." Paul McCartney

This new way of life for me has some scientific origin because many studies have shown that a calorie restricted diet contributes greatly to a healthier body as well as to longevity. A calorie is a calorie, yes but the quality of foods is the key contributor. Anyone would lose weight by burning more calories than they consume but it is important to remember that if you are going to reduce caloric intake, to consume quality nutrient rich calories. The foods you consume can vary significantly from day to day, so it does not have to be a mundane task. Mix up what you eat and discover new all natural foods that you will enjoy.

To reiterate, I have always been a healthy minded person but consciously I decided that I wanted to be thinner as I age. I want to give my body and mind a better chance of longevity and quality of living.

As I remember back in my life, I felt best at 160 pounds and I guess that is why I have that figure in mind. At 5'10" I am medium built and at 53 I do not need any extra weight to carry around. I do not fear death, but I do fear aging ungracefully. Aging ungracefully is no way to live. Our society has come to expect certain diseases to accompany aging, but this does not have to be the norm. It is not the norm in cultures that eat lower on the food chain and get regular exercise.

Summary from day 47:

30 ounce carrot, apple, beat, gingery and celery juice: 450

Large mixed salad: 400

Total calories: 850

Exercise: 15 mile bike ride. 75 push-ups and sit-ups.

Thoughts from my bike ride: I rode my bicycle by a Walgreens today and noticed a long line at the pharmacy drive-thru and couldn't help but think, "How many of those people would not need "their pills" if they would commit to a plant based diet? Let us say, for argument sake, that 25% could get off all medications as a result. That is still a lot! Imagine the enhancement of their lives, the increased quality and the joy they would experience to avoid all those side effects of drugs? Imagine the cost savings to them and the entire health care system? The list goes on!

However, does not it behoove pharmaceutical companies for people to be sick? More profit, right? Isn't it possible, because of decreased profits, that hospitals, the meat industry, the dairy industry and processed food industries would not welcome the change in food consumption that I propose?

DAY: 48

WEIGHT: 182
DATE: SEPTEMBER 13, 2016

"Even as a junkie I stayed true [to vegetarianism] - 'I shall have heroin, but I shan't have a hamburger.' What a sexy little paradox." Russell Brand

I find the above quote funny as it hits home because at one point in my early 20s, I was snorting cocaine, taking a few pills and drinking a little too heavy. But at the same time, I was eating a totally vegetarian diet. I thought I would bring that out in the open because I am attempting to be brutally honest and make a point that I am hardly superior to anyone and certainly have had my share of adversity.

As early as I can remember I always had a connection to animals, the sun and nature. I remember bringing home stray dogs, talking to birds and thinking they talked back. So, yea, you could say, as my mother used to, that I was an odd kid. But from my perspective, a respect for animals did not take much effort, it just was. However, I can imagine for some it is difficult to correlate a love for animals and eating them at the same time. I must remind myself that giving up meat is not so easy for most of the people in America. Hopefully, I can sway a few with this book.

Many Americans sit all day at an office or break their backs at a construction site, etc., so it is important to feed the body good fuel and take time out of your day for walking, bike riding, running or whatever you enjoy. And if you are older, I think aging people need to play by different rules than the young. We need to be more conscious of everything we do. Or we can simply buy in to the bullshit about aging and the "that's just the way it is attitude" and choose to take pills to lower our cholesterol and blood pressure. We can accept our low blood sugar and diminished sex drive.

Summary from day 48:

20 ounce carrot, beet, ginger, celery and apple juice: 375

16 ounce banana and strawberry smoothie: 300

Some potato chips and a soy bologna sandwich: 500

Total calories: 1175

Exercise: 20 mile bike ride. 40 push-ups.

Thoughts from my bike ride: As we age, let us say past 40, its time we think about eating a gentle diet (and eat less) if we expect longevity and graceful aging. Our metabolic rate slows down after 40 and it is no secret that all kinds of ailments will creep in if you let it.

DAY: 49

WEIGHT: 182
DATE: SEPTEMBER 14, 2016

"Very occasionally, if you pay really close attention, life doesn't suck." Joss Weldon

What we eat, without question, affects our happiness. Detrimental foods can contribute greatly to low self-esteem, lack of energy, sex drive and disease. But this does not have to be the case. Change the way you eat and change your life! It is that simple for most. Stop eating shit and start living again!

In our middle aged years, it seems that much of our socializing revolves around food. We get asked to dinner regularly or stay at home and make large meals. We crave sweets and fast food because our bodies are crying out to feel good, even though that relief we get from junk food is very temporary. Is this how it is supposed to be, one will ask himself? But when you turn it around and start eating whole-plant based foods, you will find that you do not really crave anything but good foods that quench your natural hunger. The interesting part is, these foods you will now desire, if you adopt a plant based diet, will satisfy you thoroughly, unlike the guilt that accompanies a quick fix of ice cream or cheesecake.

What people eat does not make them a good or bad person. I have some friends that do not even know I am a health minded person, who devour many high fat- meat based meals right before my eyes but I do not judge them. The food choices we make can be changed at any time and many times the "why" we eat what we do is a subconscious decision that we consciously are not aware of. Advertising and childhood reward systems is the culprit but that is just a glimpse in to "the why."

So how can we expect to age gracefully? One could spend less time in the car, get a different job, live on less, demand "time out" for exercise at work, eat lunch at a juice bar, kill your TV, buy a bike and keep only whole foods at your house. Move to a warmer climate in a smaller house with no television. Live closer to work and use public transportation. It is your choice, isn't it?

Summary from day 49:

Raw cucumbers, broccoli and celery: 300

16 ounce carrot, lime, beet and apple juice: 300

Vegetarian hot and sour soup with rice: 500

Total calories: 1100

Exercise: 11 mile bike ride. 50 push-ups.

Thoughts from my bike ride: For many Americans, the reality is that they drive an hour in a metal coffin (cars) to spend 8 hours in a toxic office. As a result, it becomes a difficult task prioritizing food choices. Its just to easy to go buy food at a drive-through. Just being aware of this fact can promote change.

DAY: 50

WEIGHT: 181
DATE: SEPTEMBER 15, 2016

"After all, tomorrow is another day." Margaret Mitchell

I keep telling myself to take this one day at a time and stay the course. Although it has been easier than I thought I do have moments where I see pizza and I wish it were actually good for me. But for the most part I do not feel deprived. To the contrary, I feel satisfied and very much sustained.

I am excited that I have only 10 days to go before I start to wrap up this book. I am hopeful I will be down to 175 by that time (I was shooting for 160 to 170). However, if I fall short, no big deal. Eventually I will reach my goal of 160 pounds and stay there (or below) until leaving this body.

According to most weight charts I am still overweight. Most have me between 145 and 170 pounds as being ideal. But many men, especially men, say that they do not feel comfortable when they lose too much weight. It is my belief that this is due to mind implant systems from male macho authority figures who imbed these petrified opinions into young male minds. The reason this exist, in my opinion, is due to men wanting to be muscular and big because they see that as the benchmark from youth. It is much like woman having a tainted self-image that they need to be thinner and have big boobs. Fact is, many weightlifters are overweight, despite their pleasing visual appearance. As we age, it is ever more important to reduce body weight in which will greatly increase organ function and add years to one's life.

Summary from day 50:

20 ounce lemon, carrot, beet, ginger and celery juice: 350

2 black bean burgers (no bread): 400

Large mixed salad: 350

Total calories: 1100

Exercise: 16 mile bike ride. 50 push-ups.

Thoughts from my bike ride: Today I was people watching as I rode my bike. I could not help but notice that most of the walkers, runners and bikers were tuned in to some sort of music devise, texting, looking at social media or talking on the phone. In my humble opinion, I think exercise should be a form of meditation and you cannot mediate when you are still plugged in. Exercise is a great time to work things out! Thus- for me anyway, I unplug for those moments and become one with nature for just a bit. Yet another reason why I prefer biking and outdoor exercise over a gym. There are too many loud noises and distractions at most gyms but to each his own.

DAY: 51

WEIGHT: DID NOT WEIGH IN
DATE: SEPTEMBER 16, 2016

"Nature itself is the best physician." Hippocrates

As the above quote postulates, you must get in tune with nature and its plethora of cures available to you. Eating a plant based diet is a good start. Modern medicine excels when it comes to fixing broken bones, surgery, etc. but it is not always the answer to internal issues that can be cured with proper nutrition.

As I watch baseball on television tonight, I am being bombarded with so called food commercials that insinuate that their clients poison will give me immense joy. Worst yet, some advertisers pray on children and you cannot help but notice the racial connotations as well. As an example-observe how many African Americans are given parts in McDonald's, Popeye's and Kentucky Fried Chicken commercials. It is ironic that African Americans suffer amongst the highest rates of heart disease and diabetes. This is an outrage to me and grossly irresponsible.

Fast food restaurants are a major factor in destroying our people. It even reaches to China, were the Chinese used to enjoy superior health but that is not the case today due to fast food chains bullying their way into those societies and addicting the people. How is this not worst than all drug dealers combined? There is no doubt in my mind that soon China will suffer the consequences of this dietary change.

There are many diets that can help you lose weight, but all have something similar. And that is, reduction of caloric intake. I have tried all kinds of diets from high protein to anything you can imagine but this modified fast, infused with micronutrient rich easily assimilated foods has proven its superiority to me. The weight loss has been nice but the healing of my skin and sharpness of my mind has me convinced.

Charles Caprarella

Summary from day 51:

Large bowl of brown rice and vegetables: 500

20 ounce carrot, beet, ginger, apple and cucumber juice: 350

Tomato soup and corn: 350

Total calories: 1200

Exercise: 12 mile bike ride. 25 push-ups.

Thoughts from my bike ride: When I was a kid growing up in the 70s my dad had his first heart attack at only 39. Animal foods, along with smoking clogged his arteries, as was said by his cardiologist. I think this event had an impact on me and solidified what I always thought, "why do people eat animals?"

I thought at the time that by the time I was 40 that probably 80% of the world would be vegetarian because of progress. However, the meat and dairy industry, along with advertisers did their job by spending billions to make sure that did not happen. Now, at 53, extraordinarily little progress has been made. In fact, we have gone progressively backwards. But I am hopeful that a crusade will begin and in 20 years eating animals will be a thing of the past.

DAY: 52

WEIGHT: DID NOT WEIGH IN
DATE: SEPTEMBER 17, 2016

"Let your food be your medicine, and your medicine be your food." Hippocrates

I find advertisements representing pharmaceutical companies sneaky and insulting to our intelligence. The hired advertising agencies use good looking actors to portray joy that will accompany their client's drug use. As if by taking these drugs, that everything will be alright! Ironically, and not by accident, immediately following these drug commercials, there are food advertisements- pushing their product on you that are largely responsible for you having to take pills in the first place. Thus, we can safely conclude that the "system" is all connected, that it wants us sick and addicted?

How do we counter those brainwashing images we get bombarded with when we watch television? I guess for one, do not watch it and simply be aware of the reality of it. Start eating a whole food-plant based diet and do not allow the medical establishment to dictate your course of action. Yes, modern medicine can be a good partner in healing but many times you can help heal yourself by eating properly.

Pharmaceutical companies have used advertising to manipulate Americans for years. They want you to feel safe, knowing that their drugs will cure you. That ailments are just part of aging. Have diabetes? Take a pill! Have high cholesterol? Take a pill!

If you want to age gracefully with honor, put aside the knives and use forks instead. Eating low on the food chain is your responsibility to yourself and future generations.

The Native American's looked to the elders for wisdom about various topics ranging from love, health and life. However, many of our elderly today have much to offer but how to eat is not one of them. Instead, our elderly line-up at restaurants, coupons in hand, and gorge on processed foods on a regular basis. We aging people need to become examples to our youth, like the proud healers of the original residents of America!

Summary from day 52:

16 ounce apple, carrot, ginger and beet juice: 300

16 ounce banana and strawberry smoothie: 300

Small salad: 200

Bag of potato chips: 200

Total calories: 1000

Exercise: 12 mile bike ride. 100 push-ups. 60 sit-ups.

Thoughts from my bike ride: Eating this way is giving me a deeper connection with Mother Earth and her healing foods!

DAY: 53
WEIGHT: 180
DATE: SEPTEMBER 18, 2016

"If you are not your own doctor, you are a fool." Hippocrates

We are so fortunate to be alive during this era of technology where one can easily enter a subject in to a search field and research any subject. Personally, I do not think the academics of the world, including doctors, lawyers and teachers always appreciate this ability because for the first time in the history of the world they are being questioned at an unparalleled level.

We have all heard the statement, "everyone thinks they are an expert now because of the internet." Although, I agree with this to an extent, many people have benefited greatly from internet research and application. The bottom line is, at no other time in the history of the world has the common man been on such an even playing field with the academic community. But this is a threat to the academic community because knowledge was once protected by the institutions that felt it was proprietary and the only way they would share is for one to attend those institutions that housed the books and professors to share it.

One could say that Google and YouTube, to name a few, has had more significant impact on knowledge than all schools combined. We enter a new age, and it is the age of enlightenment. As we become our own best doctors, we will become more of a threat to the profit margins of the meat, dairy and food processors of the world. As we start to heal from the whole-plant based foods that we now consume, hospital parking lots will start to become empty and the legal drug pushers will start to fold. Health insurance will become a brutally competitive field that offers affordable pricing and alternative treatments to its customers. Additionally, advertisers will no longer be able to push their death foods on the public for profit. You see, becoming healthy is good for you but not good for multitudes who have become comfortable making millions off demised health.

Summary from day 53:

16 ounce carrot, ginger, beet and cucumber juice: 300

Veggie burger: 350

Vegetarian hot and sour soup and rice: 600

Total calories: 1250

Exercise: 10 mile bike ride. 75 push-ups.

Thoughts from my bike ride: As I rode my bike at the local park today, I enjoyed the mild weather, but I could not help but notice the many groups of people grilling. As I got closer, I looked to see what was being served. Hamburgers, barbeque chicken, potato salad, chips, soda and hot dogs was amongst all groups but one. That group was an Indian family that was serving a wide variety of deliciously smelling dishes and no grilling. I grew saddened as I envisioned the inevitable diminished health of the frequent consumers of grilled meats.

DAY: 54

WEIGHT: 180
DATE: SEPTEMBER 19, 2016

"If you want to live a happy life, tie it to a goal, not to people or things." Albert Einstein

When I started this book, my goal was to get down to 160 to 170 pounds within 60 days. Right now, I weigh 180. It has been a long time since I have been 180 but when I lived in New Mexico from 1990 to 2001 I weighed anywhere from 160 to 170 and felt comfortable at that weight. I felt like that was my ideal weight. I was running 3 to 5 miles a day, lifting weights, biking and swimming too. I was eating way too much food, but the excessive exercise allowed me to eat whatever I wanted, and I was still able to maintain my weight. I felt good but in the long-run that is an unhealthy way to live as the body never gets a break from digesting food. But some people live a lifestyle that require a high caloric intake, such as a football player or marathon runner, etc.

I absolutely love life and all that it offers so I figure why not try and get the absolute best out of it. Reducing caloric intake and eating highly nutritional food is a great way to improve the quality of life. There is literally no other better statistically proven way to accomplish healthy longevity.

I have lost a total of 32 pounds in 54 days and as a result I am starting to feel like my 40 year old version of me.

Where I live at this time of year, it is a common tradition for adults to spend the weekends drinking a lot of beer, watching football on the tube and eating the foods that are advertised during those football games. Pizza, chips, Doritos and grilled meats are the main course. Thus- it is no coincident that many middle aged people that I know take pills to lower "their" high blood pressure, control their diabetes and lower their cholesterol. This is their normal!

We are pawns to the NFL and all television shows! Their very existence is designed to get you to watch so that their paying advertisers can brainwash your mind. As a result, we pollute our bodies with their products and the consequences are eventual suffering and early death.

Imagine for a moment that brown rice and carrot juice was offered at a baseball game instead of beer and hot dogs being the norm. You just cannot eat or drink too much of those items. As a result, there would not be much profit in it. However, we would all be happier, healthier and kinder to the planet.

Do not get me wrong, many people do not even watch sports and are extremely active but what I am saying is that what I have described is quite common. It is simply not worth it to feel good in "the now", for a moment, and suffer unspeakable extended periods of suffering in the future.

Football season goes on for months leading all the way up to the Super Bowl so this punishment to the body goes on month after month and in some cases, year after year. But it gets worst. Not only does this time of year offer football but the holidays as well. We cram bad food in our body's right up until New Years and it seems as though we enjoy this practice.

We are like zombies to the food and drug companies and then we wait until New Years to proclaim our wish to lose weight for the upcoming year. Pure insanity if you ask me!

Nobody could, if honest, tell me that going for a long walk on a nice day and eating healthy foods is not more fulfilling than drinking beer all day and eating poison. If that is a preferred activity you are kidding yourself and assuredly you will be wanting a time machine when the inevitability of early sickness and disease sets in. In short, it is not worth the cheap high you get in the now, compared to the suffering you will experience in the future. Heart disease, diabetes, obesity, arthritis, nursing homes, surgeries, sexual dysfunction, cancer and many other ailments are all largely a result of the lifestyle choices one has been making for many years.

For the most part, we are all created equal biologically and we react like the fuel (food) that we put in our bodies so why not choose good fuel that plant based foods will provide you? Yes, genetics play a role but not as much as you might think. Most studies show that 70% of all sickness is a simple lifestyle choice. The "what to eat" debate can be a life or death choice and or one of popping pills and disease. Each time you choose good foods you are choosing a life of robust living!

It is no accident that NFL football games are enamored with Viagra and Cialis commercials as well. Sexual dysfunction has been shown to be largely a result of what you eat and the pills you pop, not the normal aging process of men. When you think about it, it is absurd how many men over 40 take a pill to function in the bedroom! When you get down to it, football, food, pills and sexual dysfunction are largely connected.

However, it could be that we spend our weekends at the opera, going to plays and visiting art museums and for lunch we have a wonderful lobster casserole and steak dinner? But many times, these presumably more cultured actives can have deadly consequences as well. Because many of these foods are horridly destructive to our bodies. Animal foods can be beautifully prepared but at the end of the day they are no better for you than a big mac.

I am no better than anyone and my behavior is hypocritical at times. I like to smoke cigars and from time to time have caved in and ate an entire bag of chips. My point is, as we age, we need to know what drives us before we can begin to change. I do not intend to quit drinking or give up cigars, but I am not going to kid myself and live a lie.

Food is everyone's problem as it effects the animals, the environment, our health care system and the future of the planet.

Summary from day 54:

30 ounce banana, strawberry and orange smoothie: 400

Huge mixed salad: 450

Almonds: 400

Total calories: 1250

Exercise: 14 mile bike ride. 40 push-ups. 40 sit-ups.

Thoughts from my bike ride: We often hear people say, "They would trade all the money in the world for good health." When people are diagnosed with an illness you would expect more would quit their jobs, mortgage their house, move to a warmer climate, buy a bike and trade in knives for forks. But to the contrary, many elect surgery and pills. They keep working long hours and eat comfort foods.

Let us re-examine. When people say, "They would trade all the money in the world for good health," they are really talking about when they are on their death beds. But that is a little too late, isn't it so? So, let us imagine another world. You go to the doctor's office and get diagnosed with a bad illness such as heart disease, diabetes or cancer. The doctor quickly prescribes a juice fast for 30 days and then directs you to eat raw whole foods for the rest of your life. He tells you to quit your stressful job, make life simpler, buy a bike and move to a warmer climate. He tells you <u>to</u> start investing that money you saved for better health. Witch scenario would you choose?

In scenario number 2 you could grow older with dignity. You would be kinder to the environment and animals. You will not become a burden on our failing health care system. When you die, it is with dignity and fight!

DAY: 55

WEIGHT: DID NOT WEIGH IN
DATE: SEPTEMBER 20, 2016

"Don't waste your energy trying to change opinions ... Do your thing, and don't care if they like it." Tina Fey

I have heard many opinions as to what the right diet is or is not and I have been criticized over many years for being a vegetarian and there may be some truth to things. However, I have read many books, watched documentaries and have experimented on myself so I am confident it is a good choice. At the end of the day, I listen to my instinct and you just cannot please everyone.

I am not happy with myself for getting over 200 pounds. But I have done something about it by acting and that I feel good about. For me, weight gain has always been easy and when I was younger it would come off faster but now at 53 it takes more effort.

Thinner people appear to eat better than heavier people but many times this is not the case. What I am saying is, sometimes your apparent curse is your blessing and vice versa. Many people who are naturally thin do not feel like they have the need to count calories nor eat healthy. Hopefully, I am making my point here. So thin people truly must think beyond what they see in the mirror and eating healthy is harder for them. We have all known people that eat what they want and do not gain an ounce. Anyway, being the way I am, easy to gain weight, has afforded me the opportunity to try harder and think deeply.

As I exercised today, I realized that my hour long or so bike rides only burn about 400 calories and that is equivalent to not much food by today's standards. We humans must be designed to eat less food than we do because it seems so easy to take in calories but harder to burn them. Thus- the only logical answer is that our current standards for caloric intake are too high.

Summary from day 55:

20 ounce banana, strawberry, pineapple and orange smoothie: 350

Vegetarian minestrone soup: 400

Some whole grain bread: 200

Total calories: 950

Exercise: 11 mile bike ride. 50 push-ups. 30 sit-ups.

Thoughts from my bike ride: I shopped at a Fresh Thyme supermarket today with my daughter and ended up eating some delicious vegetarian minestrone soup and some multi grain bread. It was a good day with her, and I was pleasantly surprised at the healthier food choices. Still though, the shelves in this so called healthy market are packed with processed foods, albeit at a better level than a traditional market, nonetheless, processed. And I was sickened by the number of meats not only sold but marketed as "all natural". Everywhere we turn, we are being "sold".

So called healthy markets do their best but beware of the manipulation to make one feel healthier or superior in their marketing. When you walk in these places, its best to go right to the bulk food section and then over to the produce section and then get the hell out. It is far too easy to be suckered in to buying a bunch of processed foods.

DAY: 56

WEIGHT: 179
DATE: SEPTEMBER 21, 2016

"A journey of a thousand miles begins with a single step."
Lao Tzu

This 60 day experiment of mine; reducing calories, losing weight and eating only whole-plant foods has a destination but it will not be over when I arrive. At times I will fall short, but this will be my benchmark for the rest of my life.

Multitudes of conclusive studies has shown that a long-term calorie restricted diet is an ideal way to achieve good health and longevity. Of course, there are no guarantees but there are many other reasons to live on less food as well.

One must just sit outside of a McDonalds (not to pick on them) and observe to realize that food addiction, without question, is a bigger problem than all drug addictions combined. Food addiction is silent, and it masks itself well with pretty packaging as it slowly kills us. It does and not impair one's ability to drive or operate heavy machinery. It is a slow killer!

We all have addictions to something or another and let me be clear, I am no better than anyone else. I have had times in my life that I got addicted to this or that. As an example, I like my morning coffee and have a hard time functioning without it.

It is not my point to belittle anyone. My point is, that we need to be enlightened to the fact that many so called foods have become an addiction and is slowly killing us and our planet. Minimizing our consumption of all foods and replacing processed foods with mostly plant based foods is the cure. I use the word minimize to leave room for error. The universe is not perfect, nor are we.

Summary from day 56:

20 ounce carrot, ginger, beet, lime and apple juice: 350

Vegetable fajita: 400

Wheat pasta with spinach and tomato: 350

Total calories: 1100

Exercise: 11 mile bike ride. 25 push-ups. 25 sit-ups.

Thoughts from my bike ride: I only have 4 more days before I start to wrap up this book and I am ready. I have gone long enough to experience great results and the way I feel is extraordinary. Father time has turned back 15 years!

DAY: 57

WEIGHT: 179
DATE: SEPTEMBER 22, 2016

"The world as we have created it is a process of our thinking. It cannot be changed without changing our thinking." Albert Einstein

Good old Albert was right on target with this quote. As I was eating my vegetable fajita last night, out to dinner with a friend, my good friend was especially combative. He said, "You know, having just a little bit of junk food is not a bad thing and plenty of people eat all natural meat." So, I said, "There is nothing natural about meat and I doubt very much they only eat "all natural meat", because it is availably is so scarce, and besides, there is nothing natural about eating animals. If it were natural, why wouldn't we mount a cow and bite its neck when we are hungry? Why is it we prepare it carefully, cut its head off and cook it? Most likely it is so we will not have to look at its eyes. Eyes are said to be the window of the soul so when we eat something with eyes, we are essentially eating everything it has experienced." I continued to say, "We are omnivores", but he said, "That cavemen ate dinosaurs."

I know he was kidding about the dinosaurs, maybe, but why is it we want to eat like a caveman or for that matter follow a caveman's advice?

The Paleo Diet, also called the Caveman Diet, is a diet consisting of supposedly what earlier humans ate. Yes, it is good in premise because no processed foods were around back then. However, earlier humans hardly had the luxuries that we have, nor the choices. To add, our animals of today are factory raised, packed with hormones, steroids, antibiotics and suffer unspeakable torture before death. Furthermore, we now know in this overpopulated world of 9 billion people that consciously we cannot continue to ravish the world of the resources it takes to feed people animals. It is really a bogus argument from many levels.

Earlier hunters and gatherers ate whatever they could find! So where does one go with a conversation like that, I thought? This is a good friend, so I shut up and tried to change the subject. Unfortunately, though, diet talk can be much like political and religious talk as many times it can get "heated". Everyone wants to be right, voices raise, and any sense of reasoning and rational thought can go out the window fast.

For most animals that are served on a plate or in burger bun, their life was one of torture, mutilation, darkness and suffering. Its very death was its only joy!

He continued, "How do you know that eating meat is not good for us and many people live long lives eating meat and many thin people that are vegetarians die young." I tried to explain statistics, studies, cultures, mounting evidence, the history of economics, advertisers, lobbyist and that body weight does not tell the entire story. That thin people can be unhealthy and larger people can be healthy. I even tried to explain how eating meat greatly contributes to the destruction of earth and that there is widespread animal torture in the meat production business, but I wasn't getting anywhere.

These conversations are difficult ones because I know deep down, I am on target, but one can easily come across as a "know it all" so sometimes its best, for sake of friendship and sanity to just placate to others and save it for another day or in this case, write a book. I figure when people read this book there will be much criticism and maybe I might lose a few friends but that is the risk I am willing to take.

Summary from day 57:

40 ounce carrot, apple, beet and ginger juice: 600

Veggie burger: 400

Eggplant and vegetable dish: 300

Total calories: 1300

Exercise: 12 mile bike ride. 50 push-ups.

Thoughts from my bike ride: I cannot shake the conversation I had with my friend last night. I feel bad we had a heated argument about the effects of food and how silly that was.

Many times, I feel so alone in this quest, that I am some sort of freak or something but since an incredibly young age, I have known that it was my calling to help people rid themselves of eating animals and for animals to live a free life, void from the cold hearts of humans.

DAY: 58

WEIGHT: 178
DATE: SEPTEMBER 23, 2016

"Have no fear of perfection - you'll never reach it." Salvador Dali

The reason why I estimated my caloric intake is that seeking perfection is impossible. Although, having a basic knowledge of caloric intake of foods is a must. Set a calorie max for each day and try not to exceed it. But if you do exceed those number, do not worry about it and try harder the next day.

I have been living well on less than 1200 calories a day. I am sure I could eat more than that but that would require more exercise and activity to maintain or lose weight. Besides, eating less is gentle on your body, the planet and you can maintain weight with extraordinarily little effort.

Although, anyone could easily eat 5000 calories a day and maintain or even lose weight if they are continually active. But what I am doing is for the common man- the 80% of the population who just want to live a healthy life.

This diet choice is not for the young, the ultra-thin nor a person with an eating disorder. This diet is for most of the population who suffer with overeating and unwanted weight.

Summary from day 58:

16 ounce apple, carrot and beet juice: 300

Almonds: 200

Large salad: 400

Vegetable soup: 300

Total calories: 1200

Exercise: 11 mile bike ride.

Thoughts from my bike ride: I have decided to completely fast for the last two days of this journal before I wrap up this book. I figure it is a good way to end it.

DAY: 59

WEIGHT: 178
DATE: SEPTEMBER 24, 2016

"The power of fasting is miraculous." Lailah Gift Akita

As I get ready to end my journal of 60 days, I feel it appropriate to eat little for the next couple of days. I have lost over 30 pounds and I feel as though my addiction to food is curbed but hardly over. I was able to re-program my mind on a plant based-whole food diet-consisting of mostly raw foods, but I am sure I will be tempted again.

I have enjoyed juicing both vegetables and making fruit smoothies so much that I intend to make it part of my life, although not a regimen. Juicing gives the body an immediate lift and it has no crash or bad side effects.

I do not intend to keep a written journal of the foods I consume any longer, as I feel like I can keep a running total in my mind for now. I intend to weigh myself one a week or so.

This is my new way of life and I look forward to a compromised free life. At least a life free from food addiction. I wish you the same too.

Summary from day 59:

1 apple: 125

1 banana: 175

Total calories: 300

Exercise: 13 mile bike ride.

Thoughts from my bike ride: Today was a pleasant ride, knowing I am one day away from finishing this journal.

DAY: 60
WEIGHT: 176
DATE: SEPTEMBER 25, 2016

"Life is at its best when everything has fallen out of place, and you decide that you're going to fight to get them right, not when everything is going your way and everyone is praising you."
Thesauri Wanniarachchi

Moving to Indiana might have been my destiny because if I had stayed in New Mexico I probably would have never fallen out of place, but the future is bright and without the experience I might have never written this book. So hopefully a few people benefit and change their lives for the better, as a result of reading it.

A study by Jonathan Tilly of Harvard Medical School, shows that reducing the caloric intake of older mice by 40 percent significantly reduces the number of eggs with abnormal chromosomes. A similar study by Tilly concluded that restricting food intake of adult mice extended their reproductive lifespan and the health of their offspring. Studies on the benefits of fasting span back thousands of years and are backed up by many scientific studies so why not give it a try? Best of luck!

Summary from day 60:

1 apple: 150

Small salad: 200

Total calories: 350

Exercise: 15 mile bike ride. 100 push-ups.

Thoughts from my bike ride: I am excited to have finished this book. And I hope you have enjoyed it. Additionally, I have included some additional thoughts for you.

Steps we can take to lose weight and live life to the fullest:

- Eliminate all animal foods
- Kick start your bodies healing process with a 14 day juice fast
- Throw away all processed food in your house
- Consult a doctor if you take pills and have known health issues
- Start to exercise
- Keep a journal
- Eat at least 60% of foods, raw
- Read a book a month about health, start with Diet for a New America
- Base socializing around less food
- Watch videos on how to prepare raw healthy foods
- Plan ahead when going out to dinner and healthier restaurants
- Watch less TV
- Question doctors, teachers and parents
- Seek alternative treatments
- Consider a smaller refrigerator or get rid of it
- Consider moving to a warmer climate
- Try to meet more like-minded people
- Buy a bike
- Demand exercise rooms at work
- Park further away
- Walk over driving
- Do what it takes to be healthier
- Make your own list

Feel free to contact me anytime by text or email:
Charles Caprarella, 317-319-2365 or ccaprarella@aol.com

In the following pages, I am going to share some thoughts that have helped me live a more enriched life:

EXERCISE

"Waking is man's best medicine." Hippocrates

They did not have bicycles thousands of years ago nor elaborate weight rooms, but they obviously had learned over time that healthy people tended to stay busy by keeping one foot in front of the other.

In John Robbins great book Healthy at 100, his research follows 4 cultures that have experienced exceptional health and longevity for thousands of years and without question, walking (staying busy) is at the forefront of the reasons why. I highly recommend reading this detailed book about health and longevity.

To me exercise is mental therapy as well as physical and cannot be avoided. I started consistently riding a bicycle, swimming, running and weightlifting 28 years ago and have not stopped since. Today, as I am older, I mostly ride my bike and lift weights. During exercise, it is a great time to think and work things out in your head.

For me, I find it best to have no music and I like to be alone or with a quiet person. I tune out from electronics so that my mind has full focus to problem solve and feed itself. It is sort of like changing the oil in my car. Every exercise session makes me feel replenished.

There are so many books and theories about exercise that your head will spin. Keep it simple and find what works for you but make no excuses and just do it!

But I will say that I think it is important to find an exercise program that emphasizes being outside instead of inside. Being outside with nature will start to reacquaint you with your synchronicity with the universe.

You hardly must become a body builder or a triathlete to reap the benefits of exercise, nor spend thousands of dollars on equipment, trainers and a gym membership. It is your divine right to be fit and it does not have to cost anything.

The benefits of exercise are well documented, and you will rarely get an argument from anyone on this subject so why don't we all do it? It takes some will power and the "path to least resistant" is a human flaw we all possess. It is a lot easier to watch TV or take a nap. Therefore, mental exercise is just as important. One feeds the other, physical and mental are in sync together.

Do the best you can and take it slow at first, but I guarantee you that you will not ever regret it afterwards. Exercise is your first path to enlightenment. Think of it like breathing, it's something you have to do.

JUDGMENT FREE

"Who are you to judge the life I live. I know I am not perfect and don't live to be but before you start to point fingers make sure your hands are clean." Bob Marley

You will find this to be the most difficult task of all for "judgment" surrounds us like the very air we breathe, and it comes from parents, teachers, loved ones, friends, foes, TV, media, books, everywhere!

It amazes me that some of the most judgmental people are also deeply religious. This startles me because the "holy books" are chalk- full of non-judgmental quotes. I often wonder, are people just not listening at their church? The truth is that being judgmental shows others that you are insecure in your belief systems.

Start this journey by trying to go hours without judgment, then an entire day and you will start to see and feel a positive transformation. You will feel better about yourself and free up your mind from this useless mind poison that all of us have become victim to.

My mother used to say, "If everyone swept their own front steps the world would be clean".

I think this is true mentally as well as physically. Imagine a world where judgment was the exception to the rule, but this must start with you. It is a most difficult task and sometimes you almost must duct tape over your mouth, but it is well worth it.

I am not suggesting you do not have an opinion and become some sort of smiling fool. I am suggesting you free yourself of useless judgment of others that have no bearing on your life this way or that way. Free up your mind of evil judgment and simply refuse to participate in conversations that involve judgment. Change the subject, politely leave the room or defuse these cancer conversations with humor.

For me, I remind myself everyday with the use of affirmations and now every time the judgment starts in conversations, my subconscious kicks in and I am now extremely sensitive to it. After time, you will see yourself start to become the person that puts out judgment fires, instead of starting them.

EAT LOW ON THE FOOD CHAIN

"You put a baby in a crib with an apple and a rabbit. If it eats the rabbit and plays with the apple, I'll buy you a new car."
Harvey Diamond

I first became I vegetarian at 12 out of sheer disgust. I watched a documentary on slaughterhouses and I just could not eat meat anymore. I had no clue that it was better for me, I just had an epiphany that it was not right.

I started eating a little meat again during my late teen years until about 25 and then I read the book Diet for a New America by John Robbins and I was done for good.

It's no secret that eating lower on the food chain is a better choice for our bodies and our environment, but this is easier said than done in this world of fast food chains, romantic advertisers, food pyramids and a plethora of opinions hitting us in every direction.

I can tell you eating little meat in my life has worked out terrific for me. I have not been sick in many years and enjoy solid health and I assure you I have never experienced the "protein myth deficiency". Although, I do eat too much and am working on that.

I am not suggesting you stop eating meat immediately but research this subject, consult a nutritionist, read books and mostly listen to your inner self.

This will not be an easy task because the meat and dairy industries are powerful and have been infiltrating our minds and for years have been brainwashing teachers, doctors, parents, about the benefits of their products via TV advertising, food pyramids and manipulative studies.

For me, I find myself extremely fortunate that I live in a country and time where I even have food choices and where I can choose to eat one way or the other and choose to eat less if I want. I am very thankful for this simple choice!

LAUGHTER

"If we couldn't laugh, we would all go insane." Robert Frost

Norman Cousins, wrote about his life-long experiment: that if he laughs for twenty minutes without any reason, all his tensions disappear. His consciousness grows, the dust disappears.

Norman Cousins was given a few months to live in 1964. He had Ankylosing Spondylitis, a rare disease of the connective tissues. He was told by a doctor who was his friend that he had a 1 in 500 chance of survival. He was told to 'get his affairs in order'. But Cousins would have none of it. A journalist, he was used to research and set himself to find a solution. He read and discovered that both his disease and the medicines were depleting his body of vitamin 'C', among other things. He did three things that would be unusual today and were unheard of then.

1. He fired his doctor and left the hospital to check into a hotel. He ascertained that the cultural of defeat and over medication in the hospital was not going to be good for his health. He found a doctor who would work with him as a team member as opposed to insisting on being in charge.

2. He began to get injections of massive doses of vitamin 'C'.

3. He obtained a movie projector, no small feat in those days, and a pile of funny movies including the Marx Brothers and 'Candid Camera' shows. He spent a great deal of time watching these films and laughing. And he did not just laugh. Despite being in a lot of constant pain, he made a point of laughing until his very stomach hurt from it.

Did it work? Who knows? You should know that Cousins finally died November 30, 1990 in Los Angeles, California.

We have all heard about the health benefits of laughing and we all know that we feel good doing it, but you just can't laugh for no reason. But you can start to put yourself in situations that make you laugh.

As an example: choose comedy movies over drama or action. Go to comedy clubs, watch comedy on YouTube, etc.

As one starts to exercise, eat a holistic diet and be one with nature, the laughing will come easier and more frequent. Thus why, many good things in life come in chain reactions. Laughing is universal and it is my belief that all living creatures laugh. Have you ever played with your dog or cat and realized they were laughing? I think we all have.

DO LESS

"Fear less, hope more, Eat less, chew more, Whine less, breath more, Love more, and all good things will be yours." Swedish Proverb

Long ago I was the person who laughed at quotes, like the above. As I grew enlightened, however, I began to get clued-in and I realized I was not getting that last laugh on my out of control lifestyle. Thus, change was needed.

Doing less means having to learn one of my favorite words, NO. I say no thank you when I do not really want to do something, unless it is directed at a child or it really means something deeply to the person asking. Sacrificing your time is different than wasting it.

I loved the movie Yes Man, and it holds some truth, but the fact of the matter is, many times we stress ourselves by doing too much and being a people pleaser. Sometimes you must be a NO man!

Doing less will free up time for reading, silence and you will learn that being alone to reflect is nourishing and you will appreciate things more.

LIVE SIMPLY

"Life already has so many boundaries and pressures- why add more in the garden?" Felder Rushing

Living simpler will free you from the chains of things and give you more precious time to enjoy the truly fulfilling aspects that life has to offer.

Drive a smaller car: When you have a smaller car, you will enjoy better gas mileage, have lower maintenance cost, be kinder to the environment and it will be easier to park. I understand we have kids to cart around but you can make it work. This is not about saving money; this is about easing the load off. Simple is better.

Have smaller yards and go to the parks more: There are so many great public parks that go unutilized. When you have a smaller yard, you have more free time that you will not be spending on yard work.

Eat less: We need much less food than we think. Eating less makes you feel good and you will lose weight. You will be freeing up more food for the hungry. Eating too much never makes us feel good, always worst. Start eating less today!

Take simple vacations: It is amazing how many great places there are to visit that are close to our homes. Try and do frequent day trips and get out of the house more often. Even in cold climates, get out, dress warm and go be with nature.

Watch less TV: We get so wrapped up in TV shows and even start to emulate our favorite characters. We are all guilty of this. Allow yourself a certain amount of TV time or eliminate it all together.

Tune out of social media: I love social media like the next guy but many times I feel like I am wasting my time on this low-energy source of life.

ORGANIZATION

"Don't just declutter, de-own." Joshua Becker, clutter free with *Kids*

There have been multitudes of books written on this subject and it is crucial to get organized and it's totally in your control. It does not cost anything except a little time and elbow grease.

I constantly throw or give things away that I do not need, and I always feel a little weight lifted after. It is difficult for some at first, especially hoarders, but this practice frees your mind, organizes your thoughts and puts you in line with the universe. The universe is orderly and so should you be.

The only thing I hold on to is most pictures and books as they can be dear to your heart and they are not very bulky anyway. When your surroundings are organized so too becomes your thoughts.

I am sure you have noticed that people with a lot of things, clutter, seem chaotic and sometimes out of control. This is because we get out of tune when we are overburdened with too many things.

Start going through your home, car, office and start selling what you do not need, throw it away or give it to someone who needs it. You will feel better, guaranteed!

Treat yourself and take a mini vacation with the money you earn from a garage sale. Experiences are far more valuable than useless "things".

As an example, sell that record collection you have had for years and invest in something in the present. Discover NEW music and free up space.

ADAPTATION

"It is not the strongest or the most intelligent who will survive but those who can best manage change." Leon C. Megginson

Darwin's principle of the survival of the fittest did not mean the largest or the strongest. The one who survives is the one who has the greatest ability to adapt.

"Intelligence is the ability to adapt to change." Stephen Hawking

"One of the basic rules of the universe is that nothing is perfect. Perfection simply does not exist. Without imperfection, neither you nor I would exist." Stephen Hawking

In the book, Who Gets Sick, by Dr. Blair Justice, he states that "disease of dysfunction" is the body's way of saying we have failed to adapt or adjust. We have all known people that cannot handle change and literally get themselves sick over it.

Knock on wood, I have not been sick in over 30 years, and I think it is because I learned to turn adversity into strength through meditation and self-reflection. Now again, I am not saying I will not get sick but what I am saying is stop beating yourself up and resisting change. Embrace change and smile at it!

Some people work at the same jobs for years and are miserable at it day in and day out. They are living a life of compromise and that is no way to live. By divine right you have the right to be happy. Start today- by getting rid of that fear and trying something you have always wanted to. Be adaptable.

Your failure to adapt can cause you to lose a job, a relationship, everything. And it is all just based on fear (false evidence appearing real) of the unknown and lack of self-confidence. Thus- it is crucial to be adaptable, as the willow tree flexes with the wind, not the oak tree that is stubborn and sturdy and breaks.

Sometimes stubbornness is a great thing and there are many examples of great people who have accomplished awesome things by maintaining their ground but there are also countless tragic stories of people who refuse to adapt, refuse to change. This is the way it has always been they say. Well, guess what, they are wrong and foolish. Learn to adapt and embrace change. You can do it!

PROCRASTINATION

"Procrastination is like a credit card. It's full of fun until you get the bill." Christopher Parker

Ironically, I had almost completed this book until it occurred to me that procrastination has been a flaw in my life, and I hadn't mentioned it, so this was a late addition to the book.

I have read a few books that offer deep seeded reasons why we procrastinate but I still struggle. However- when I do not procrastinate, I feel as though I have climbed a mountain. It is sometimes literally painful for me to complete simple tasks.

In the good read, The Road Less Traveled by M. Scott Peck M.D., He explains it like this:

Delaying Gratification:

"This is the process of scheduling the pain and pleasure of life in such a way as to enhance the pleasure by meeting and experiencing the pain first and getting it over with. It is the only decent way to live. We teach children this process at a young age, 'eat your vegetables first, then you can have dessert' or 'first complete your homework then you can play'. The concept is to efficiently complete the task that is least pleasurable first,

get it out of the way. Then you will have time to focus on and enjoy what you are looking forward to. This also pertains to emotionally challenging situations."

Not to make excuses but I was never taught this balance because I was not supervised very much growing up. But I have learned to make affirmations and reminders to myself to get things done. Tasks like paying taxes, bills, meeting deadlines, etc. Since these simple tasks are mundane to me, I have chosen a career path, writing, in which I truly enjoy. I have learned to delegate to others because to this day I am a procrastinator.

Artist, as an example, traditionally are procrastinators and perhaps this is one of the reasons why they are creative, due to not being bogged down with everyday tasks of mundane life. But on the other hand, what makes an accountant effective is his ability to complete his tasks joyfully.

Bottom line is, do something you enjoy.

24 HOUR GRACE PERIOD

"The ultimate measure of a man is not where he stands in moments of comfort and convenience, but where he stands at times of challenge and controversy." MLK Jr.

When I coached baseball the influence of the above quote was at the forefront of my mind. When the shit hit the fan, I laughed it off and eased the tension with humor and positive affirmations. But this behavior is not always possible. Thus-why the 24 hour rule!

Sometimes when one is confronted, our blood pressure soars, his adrenaline rushes and her mind spins out of control. You are in a toxic state at this point so it is not wise to make rash decisions that you will regret.

When this happens, it is imperative you take a deep breath, repeat the affirmation "24 hour rule", and if possible, take no action for at least 24 hours. Mediate on the issue and after 24 hours the answers will come to you. In coaching sports, you have no such luxury and will have to be more in tune.

How many times have we overreacted only to realize later what I waste of time it was? Go for a bicycle ride, a walk, sit in silence, whatever it takes to relax and do not react too quickly to adverse situations.

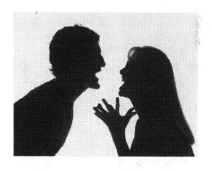

NEGATIVE PEOPLE

"Save your skin from the corrosive acids from the mouths of toxic people. Someone who just helped you to speak evil about another person can later help another person to speak evil about you." Isaelmore Avivo

To think negativity in any form is destructive to the person that cares about you most. That person is you. Think about this for a moment. You are the only one that knows exactly what you desire, so no matter what is happening around you or who is in your life, you can protect your thoughts. Simply refuse to let others get under your skin.

Make a list of these destructive people and stay away from them as much as possible. Amuse them and even manipulate them (if you are in danger) but keep a distance. This is your life, and you own it so be protective of your thoughts.

Some will think this thinking is a hocus pocus sort of new aged passing fad but its real. Take it from me, I have used this technique to help me with many adversities. It works! You will be on your road to long-lasting happiness if you apply these principles to your daily life.

Millions upon millions have found true enlightenment and so can you. If others tell you that you cannot accomplish something, run from them. It is not their life, is it? Negative people just want you to keep them company in misery. Find people that want what you want- find people of common ground.

In the wonderful booklet, ETERNAL STIMULATION ACTIVATION QUOTES, by Mystic Rose, she writes a life changing, beautiful poem:

"Let me straddle your mind...Releasing the chains that keep you blind...Catapulting your frequency within to find...You have always been free...Stop being ruled by the suppressed inner eye you refuse to see...Detach from parasitic insanity... Embrace the original ways of humanity!"

I have found it hard pressed to find people that support me, even close friends, loved ones and relatives. So I learned silence and to go about my business observing, more than talking.

I didn't really share my dream with anyone about writing this book because I am very receptive to the tonality of a person's voice, their eyes, facial expressions, etc. Many times, as we have all experienced, that's a negative karma we feel and it might stop you from moving forward with a dream.

This might be the hardest thing of all, to get away from negative people because there are so many. What works for me, is just nodding in partial agreement to avoid confrontation that will suck my vital energy sources. Sadly, most people handle disagreement aggressively. Thus- I just avoid it altogether.

Honestly, what I love about writing is, it is one sided and requires no arguments. I simply state my thoughts and you can like them or not. I am always up for a good debate, but it seems most discussion quickly turns to yelling, and it is usually not me yelling.

I once heard an Old English quote that says, "He who raises his voice first loses the argument." Unknown

So now I choose my arguments wisely and sit in silence and observe more than state my opinions. If you do this long enough you start to realize how trivial many conversations are.

On the other hand, sometimes I just think there are old souls and newer souls and that older souls cannot expect the newer souls to understand us. Some call this being enlightened, and some call it hogwash and arrogance, but I do know that sometimes you just know when I person has that twinkle in their eyes. I try being around those people as much as possible, however, you can learn much from all walks of life, if you sit and observe. Bottom line is, there is no clear cut answers, do what makes you feel good as much as possible. Listen to your instincts and hunches and never argue with those feelings.

RELIGION

"I'm not aware of too many things...I know what I know if you know what I mean...Philosophy is the talk on a cereal box... Religion is the smile on a dog." Edie Brickell

To me walking into a church is like walking in a house and never going beyond the entry way. Churches have wisdom there, as do the holy books, however, there is so much more beyond those man-made lock-step ways. I outgrew "the church" many years ago as I stepped outside the box of religion and started to explore beyond the boundaries.

We could spend days on this subject and it is probably the most controversial subject ever to exist. What is the answer, who is right? The above song, when I first heard it, kind of made sense to me. I thought when a dog smiles, she is probably happy, and it is what we all want. So maybe when you respect all living life forms. Maybe, that is god?

For me, I was raised in a Greek Orthodox and Roman Catholic Church and have no good memories. It was dark, scary and judgmental. For many years I had horrible dreams about Jesus burning and walking a large flight of stairs to my front door. We had a wooden cross with a bloody Jesus hanging on it in our house and that thing scared the crap out of me.

I find "god" in nature and it feels and familiar. I sit in silence, meditate, read, talk to my cats and get in touch with my inner-self. This satisfies me and there are only positive side effects, and it costs no money.

Once again, I am going to quote from the booklet, ETERNAL STIMULATION ACTIVATION QUOTES, by Mystic Rose, on what she says about religion:

"Religion is a mind implant of belief systems that were forced onto most people before they ever had a chance to be in alignment with their pure essence. No matter what the religion is, I notice all the people have a void from being disconnected from their eternal source. The purpose of religion is mind control and to continuously direct the energy of the repressed entity. It's fascinating for people to claim to be messengers for "God" or doing the work of "God and yet the path never leads to people being tuned into their own inner source to cut out the middle man/manipulators.

No one can lead me to anything that I can't lead myself to. Religious people don't even look vibrant, meaning they tend to look drained, tormented and confused due to being held in a repetitive hypnosis that has created blockage/fear. Everyone is naturally supposed to be a continuous evolving entity that experiences spiritual growth spurts!"

That is an honest line to take but it takes courage and conviction. Its obvious Mystic Rose is a brave woman who knows exactly what she wants, and her mind is clear. I highly recommend reading her little booklet packed with good stuff!

PASSION IN YOUR WORK

"Don't just give up trying to do what you really want to do. Where there's love and inspiration, I don't think you can go wrong." Ella Jane Fitzgerald

I was miserable as a salesman for many years but always dreamt of being a writer but just did not know how to get started so I kept reading, dreaming and having hope that one day it would just come to me and it did. And now I am a full time author and I intend to write for the rest of this life.

But it did not come easy. I just kept writing every day and things started to pull together. But we all need money so sometimes you have to do what you have to do but keep that long-term goal alive but don't ever give up your dreams. A dream is where it all begins, and you can make that dream manifest with diligent and positive thinking. Your thoughts can truly become things if you keep at it but you must practice every day, just like one would exercise physically to achieve a bodily goal. The mind requires the same.

Forthcoming so, we face many obstacles and opinions when it comes to making a living. At an early age, many times parents start to tell their little ones what they ought "to be" and this is wrong and selfish! The child implants these parental desires into their subconscious and many times spend their lives trying to please the parents, but they go about life void, making money and going to work, day after day. Therefore, I think it is crucial for parents to allow kids to follow their own path and say the words, "Do what you love and what you feel good about." We can certainly direct or advise our children, but it is wrong to direct a path.

When we graduate high school, we are expected to immediately go to college and soon after that, choose a major, a career. In lock-step conformity we march in and out of classes, many times void of any soul, desire, passion and we feel lifeless. We hear things like, "there is no money in that" and "teachers work long hours for no pay", the list goes on!

Now we graduate college or go to work, and we settle in. We become comfortable, our dreams of being an artist seem far away and unrealistic. After all, we have bills to pay and people to please. But what about us? How do we feel inside?

An Indian Guru once visited New York City and said to his guide, "what is wrong with everyone, are they being chased by wolves?" "No, said the guide, they are chasing the dollar!" Healthy At 100

Look, there are plenty of people happy at their jobs but a hell of a lot more are unhappy. So don't give up on your hopes and dreams and go for it! I am not saying to quit your job and live reckless but don't give up, even if you face opposition from loved ones. Keep pushing, keep pushing!

MIND POWER

"Belief changes the tempo for mind or thought-frequency. Like a huge magnet, it draws the subconscious forces into play, changing the whole aura and affecting everything about you-including people and objects at great distances." Claude M. Bristol

We all face enormous amounts of negative vibes from others, not just in words but in gestures that we almost must develop some sort of force field around us that protects our "space." Silence sometimes is your best shield. As an example: Do not share your dreams or desires with anyone that you know will give you a negative reaction. We all know these people! When they ask why you did not share your dream, you can politely say that it was personal to you. Guard your dreams!

When I discovered silence and mediation, it opened a world for me that was always there, but I had not yet found the doorway to it. There is no magic to this, there is no exact way to mediate. One can just sit, exist, dream and imagine the life they want. You will find that in time your desires will start to manifest for you. The Universe started with an image that manifested itself so for us, since we are all one energy, we can do the same.

I am not saying that you can become a Power Forward for the LA Lakers, because it is probably not possible physically but most things that we desire we can obtain with our thoughts. However- like any exercise, we need to be consistent. Personally, I put aside at least 1 hour a day for this. You can start with 10 minutes and gradually build but it will not be easy at first. It takes practice.

"What we believe to be true, what we believe is possible, becomes what's true, and becomes what's possible." Anthony Robbins

In Florence Scovel Shinns wonderful book The Game of Like and How to Play it, she explains it like this:

"There are three departments of the mind- subconscious, conscious and superconscious. The subconscious, is simply power, without direction. It is like steam or electricity, and it does what it is directed to do; it has no power of induction. Whatever man feels deeply or images clearly, is impressed upon the subconscious mind, and carried out in minutest detail.

The conscious mind that has been called mortal or carnal mind. It is the human mind and sees life as it appears to be. It sees death, disaster, sickness, poverty and limitation of every kind, and it impresses the subconscious.

The superconscious mind is the Divine Mind within each man, and is the realm of perfect ideas. In it, is the "perfect pattern" spoken of by Plato, The Divine Design; for there is a Divine Design for each person."

"There is a place that you are to fill and no one else can fill, something you are to do, which no one else can do." Plato

PUT SPACE BETWEEN THINGS

"Honor the space between no longer and not yet." Nancy Levin

"In that tiny space between all the givens is freedom." Sue Bender

Putting space between things means not overbooking your life, arriving early, being on-time, slowing down, not trying to do too much, etc. Just enjoying nothingness!

Learn to say NO. Learn to say no-thanks. Learn to think before agreeing to do something that you don't want to do. Think about your moments on earth as precious and maximize your time.

How many times have we all regretted saying yes to something that we were unsure about? We have all gone on those expensive-overcrowded vacations that turned into nightmares, ate unhealthy food we overpaid for, gone to movies we did not want to see, etc.? The list goes on!

I am not suggesting you become Mr. Grumpy, I am saying that a path to enlightenment cannot be cleared if you are constantly busy and not putting aside time to meditate, sit in silence and just exist with nature. This must be the main thing, not a side thing!

This is your life, and it is time to maximize your experiences and open your world to high-energy frequencies and close the door on low-energy activities that drain your soul.

Deepak Chopra, the awesome spiritual guide, explains the space between as The Gap. Below is how he is answering a question about it and I would like to share that with you. I go to the gap to free myself from fear of results.

Question: Hello Deepak I have read and still reading your book on synchronicity and seven spiritual laws. I've understood how laws work and the quantum physics as well. When I am meditating I go in the gap and then create my intent and then surrender it to the universe. I am little confused about should I be doing that every time I am meditating? Or is it something that once I surrendered then I don't create it again when am going in the gap. Unknown

Response: If you are practicing a silent meditation, then do your intentions after your meditation. Your mind will be settled in the gap, that silent state of the self. Think your intention, and then allow your awareness to be again in that silence. That is what surrendering the intention means. After a few moments, reintroduce the intention and then again let the mind return to that restful quietness. You can continue this intention practice for a few minutes, and when you are done come out as you normally would after meditation.

Love,
Deepak

"Place yourself in the middle of the stream of power and wisdom which animates all whom it floats, and you are without effort impelled to truth, to right and a perfect contentment." Ralph Waldo Emerson

I frequently take time to be one with nature. For me, I like to sit in my back yard in silence, pet cat by my side and a nice book or meditate. Whatever works for you?

If you are constantly searching for pleasure via expensive vacations, cruises, shopping-buying things, you will always be searching and never truly satisfied.

LETTING GO OF THE PAST

In Richard Carlson's (rest in peace Richard) book, Do Not Worry Make Money, there is a great story about leaving the past and the power of living in the present moment.

Imagine you are on a boat in the middle of the ocean. You are standing at the helm, heading due east, as you ask yourself three important questions: First, what is the wake? You turn back and observe the water behind the boat that is left behind. The Wake is that water. It forms a shape behind the boat until it disappears into nothingness. Second, you ask yourself the question, Can the wake drive the boat? You quickly answer, "Of course not. That's preposterous." The wake has no power. Finally, you ask yourself, what then powers the boat? You think for a moment and come to the obvious conclusion. All the power of the boat comes from the present-moment energy of the engine. That is it. There is nothing else.

This is one of the most important lessons you can activate in your life today. The past has zero power over you. Focus on what you can do today, and opportunities will come your way. Get to know yourself- look inside.

Live long and prosper!

THE END

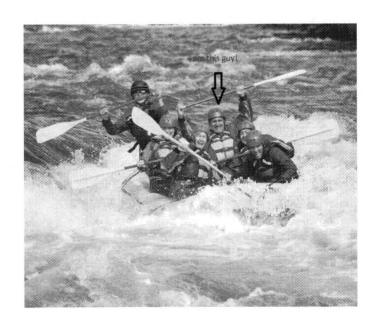

I am this guy!

Printed in the United States
by Baker & Taylor Publisher Services